Authentic Health

An Unauthorized Guide to Family Wellness

Chena Anderson ND

Authentic Health

Dedication:

This book is a product of my dedication to my children. Therefore I dedicate this work to those who both inspired and required the information contained in these pages.

To my Earthly Treasures: Christian, Felicia Joy, Charity Faith, Linnea Charrise, Liberty Grace, Solomon, Joseph, Serenity Azana-Jewel and Pneuma Flame. Each of them taught me many of the lessons shared in this life work.

For many people children are seen as something that ties you down or binds you up. I have felt this way at times, however, I encourage others to be where God has placed you in each season. Enjoy the fruits that surround you and let Him teach you the lessons that are placed in front of you through those special people in your life.

This work is the product of the lessons those people have taught me through their childhood sorrows. May they be blessed with better health than I had and I pray that they will have better mentors in health than I did at their age. This will give them the advantage of health in all their pursuits.

I also wish to acknowledge my concern for the Next Generation, my children's contemporaries. Statistical evidence strongly suggests that their generation's longevity is being affected significantly by the modern

Authentic Health

diet and the modern medical paradigm. It is projected that they will die in their fifties, twenty years before our generation. While the length of life has significantly increased over the past 100 years, it is interesting to note that the quality of those advancing years has significantly declined.

Today, people are dying of complications of the very therapy that supposedly seeks to heal them. Today, most people spend their time trying to get a quick fix for their current problems. Sadly most will never be satisfied with the quick solution, because it only drags them deeper into the problematic pit.

Health like debt drags the user down a similar pit. If you first, begin to correct the problem that caused the body to begin to be over drafted, you can then begin to rebuild your body's storehouse. The logic that taking a pill which only masks the fever, the headache, the arthritis, etc implies that a bandaid will hold closed a gaping wound. It simply never addresses the cause but simply adds to the problem. Now, there is interest accruing on the original debt and the problem or cause continues unhindered and often times worse than it was before.

What is the real solution to America's health crisis? Stop taking more out than you put in, and start storing up for tomorrow. Now, I am not just referring to cash. I am referring to healthy lifestyle and nutrition. This manual will help you stack the odds in your family's favor and rebuild their current health,

Authentic Health

without destroying them in the process. Yes, I said destroying them.

In the modern medicine paradigm, doctors often profess scientific truth and superiority. Unfortunately, it rarely fills itself with common sense. How logical is it to kill the police in order to destroy the criminals? This is how the modern antibiotic therapy works. Antibiotics kill the good and the bad. Would it not be more logical to feed the police and create an environment that is not friendly to disease and bacteria? Of course, when we want to police our streets, we clean them and provide personnel to do the work of keeping order.

This book focuses on the following 4 points:

- Recovery -- from the immediate stress.
- Restoration-- of the source of the problem.
- Strategize-- to keep the body in balance and keep symptoms from occurring again.
- Obedience – to the key principles of health.

We must first recover what has been lost. Next, we must restore the damaged areas. In order to do this, we must have a specific strategy. Finally, we must be obedient to the strategy.

Modern insurance systems have not aided us in taking power over our health. Instead they have disempowered us from making wise decisions for ourselves. I often hear, "well my insurance will cover

Authentic Health

the drugs." Does it cover the damage the drugs do? Does it teach you how not to get sick in the first place? Of course not, as it only provides bandaids to a broken system that clearly gapes open beyond the ability of any bandaid to heal.

It is my prayer that you will discover the difference in true absolute health. I pray you will enjoy the fruits of a healthy prosperous life as you develop your strategy and live within it.

Chena Anderson ND

3 John 2

Authentic Health

Introduction

I am currently the mother of 9 children. I feel as if I have been nursing or pregnant for the past 18 years. This is actually true for the most part. My husband and I met in 1992 while we were both in the mission field. We were in a children's ministry together. We married after meeting 5 months before. We never dated until after we were married. (We did not know about courtship we just knew we wanted to spend the rest of our lives with our best friend).

We left the mission field and married. We had been married 5 months when we traveled to Mexico on an evangelistic mission outreach. Upon returning, I kept feeling worse and worse, dry heaves in the night, tired all day and just all around feeling lousy. Convinced that I had some type of parasite, I kept wishing I had taken the Black Walnut I had forgotten on the counter before the trip.

Since I had been on birth control pills, I couldn't believe that I could be pregnant. However, his name is Christian and his birth sparked the contents of this book. He is the bend in the road for me. I had already begun a health journey prior to his conception. I had started cutting a lot of red meats, soda and was gradually cutting out sugar before his birth. I had given up the use of all pharmaceutical drugs. (After having an allergic reaction to prescription drugs that set my poor health even further back.) At the sudden realization that this "parasite" was the eighteen year version, we launched into the greatest journey we ever embarked on, "Parenthood."

Authentic Health

Now, nine children later, the journey continues as we launch into the teen years. "How did this happen? Or don't I know how that happened? is probably your next question. Well, to be honest we wondered how our son came to be since at the time we had put our faith in a man- made plan called "the birth control pill." The only thing this controlled was the toxifying of my body.

The manufacturers of these wonder pills have since made public the fact that they do not prevent conception but rather prevent the already conceived or fertilized embryo from finding its natural home in the uterine wall. It gives the body a false pregnancy chemically in order to keep the body from allowing another pregnancy to occur.

God intervened in our lives and by sending our son, Christian. I often think that God sent Christian to change my plan for my life. And thus our road bent in a new direction; just as God intended.

Many of you are mothers, like me. Maybe not mothers of nine but mothers no less. This is truly the highest calling of life. To not only rock the cradle, but to rule the world through your impact on the next generation.

It was because of this next generation that I began my study in herbs and nutrition. I did not want my son and any other children to have a life built on a broken paradigm, but rather built on a strong God-designed plan. This plan included good nutrition and common sense health practices that I had not been raised with. I didn't want to have to trust the "wisdom" of chemical medicine, but rather I wanted to build on the wisdom of God and His creation.

Authentic Health

With God all things are possible. Truly, I have found this to be true. By learning more about the body and the signs of ill health's approach, I have learned to be watchful of these signs and avoid excessive exposure to events like those wonderful birthday parties that children attend or when they visit grandma's house. Limiting exposure to sources for poor eating will greatly reduce the sick days in your home. Training is ultimately the key to success, without training in breaking greedy eating habits and replacing them with that of healthy moderation in eating choices.

I am not suggesting that you hide out in the hills, but I am suggesting that prevention is the best and least expensive medicine. By spending the extra on supplements for your children and family, as well as for yourself, you can avoid the enormous headaches of doctor's visits, missed days of work and productivity as well as the dollars that run out of your budget from the "security" of having medical insurance.

My children have never seen medical doctors (except when my oldest son was circumcised). How have we done it? Simply by paying attention to the signs of approaching illness and learning the cycles of development that are normal for each child and understanding the unique constitution of each child helps greatly in recognizing their "dis-ease" progression gives you the edge so that you can head off ailments before there is a problem. The process of chronic ailments comes about first in a lack of "ease" or comfort. Therefore, "dis-ease" is simply a lack of comfort, resulting in disease which a doctor may diagnose with a latin word to describe your daily pain.

Authentic Health

Where do we begin on this journey toward health and savings. Let's begin, with the basics of good health practices, diet and nutrition, and then let's learn the signs of "dis-ease", so we can see trouble coming before it arrives.

Authentic Health

Health is a state of complete harmony of the body, mind and spirit. When one is free from physical disabilities and mental distractions, the gates of the soul open. ~B.K.S. Lyengar

Authentic Health

Table of Contents

Chapter 1 Taking Care of Dr. Mom 14

Chapter 2 Going from Here to There 30

Chapter 3 Living High or on a Higher Conscious 35

Chapter 4 The Vital Factor: Sleep..............41

Chapter 5 How to make a Healthy Baby...45

Chapter 6 Healthy Beginnings: Pregnancy, Birth And Beyond........................49

Chapter 7 Birth Stories 65

Chapter 8 Baby Troubles........................82

Chapter 9 Diet For Healthy Child............94

Chapter 10 Bowel & Digestive Health: Keys to A Peaceful Mind.............100

Chapter 11 Food Allergies & Their Effect on Daily Health 112

Chapter 12 The Respiratory System......116

Authentic Health

Chapter 13 Nervous Connections: ADD, Slow Learning, Ticks, Stuttering, Eye Sight......................129

Chapter 14 The Vaccine Connection..........138

Chapter 15 Chronic Pain and Solutions.....144

Chapter 16 Everyday Pain.........................154

Chapter 17 Fevers 164

Chapter 18 Colds 171

Chapter 19 Flus 178

Chapter 20 Virus or Bacteria 181

Chapter 21 The Skin, Eczema, Poison Ivy..188

Chapter 22 Bedwetting and UTI's..............194

Chapter 23 Weight Loss & Keys to Balanced Health................199

Chapter 24 The Home Medicine Chest. 207

Author Contact Information....................211

Chapter 1: Taking Care of Dr. Mom

This Chapter will help you:

- ✓ establish healthy priorities
- ✓ put your pie in order
- ✓ enjoy the pie you make

You can only give what you've received

As a parent, we should seek to display the best example of how to live a rich life to our children. This should be in all areas of life: moral, social, spiritual, educational, and even healthy lifestyles. It is not enough to help them stay well and not strive to show them how you did it. Our daily examples set the stage for our grand children's future. If we teach good health habits, good lifestyle habits, and healthy thinking, we will reap healthy families are generations.

I, myself, constantly must strive to meet this mark. And it is difficult at times. In fact, it is difficult daily. As I write this chapter I am up at 5:00 am to have quiet time and complete one more chapter. To do this and stay healthy, I must go to bed at 9:30 pm every night. I am by nature a night owl. I have had to make some adjustments to my

Authentic Health

habits. 11:30 pm is not a bed time if I'm going to wake up at 5:30 am and feel good all day. I have had to learn to simply leave things undone until tomorrow on many occasions. And amazingly enough, the world has not come to a screeching halt because of my unwashed dishes, or incomplete planning for some event.

To begin, taking care of Dr. Mom is simply to desire health and recovery in the planning of your day. Examine the current flow of your day. This may change suddenly or dramatically over the coming years as children's needs and schedules change. An old pattern may no longer bring you the successful day you desire. An old pattern may also, bring greater stress that your body can no longer bear.

For example, for 13 plus years, we have homeschooled our children. I woke up each day at 6:00 am and no later than 7:00 am. But normally, rising at 6:00 am I started laundry, read my Bible, had a hot cup of tea and eased into the day. By 7:00 am the children were emerging and we would have breakfast together and then clean up and then start our school day.

Now, we have returned to their homeschooling lifestyle. But for two years I only schooled my oldest son, Christian. During that season our other children must be up and out of the house to attend private school 20 minutes away by 7:30 am, everyone had to be up and moving no later than 6:30 am. It took me over three

Authentic Health

months to adjust to this because my morning quiet time had now been stolen. Plus, I was pregnant and requiring a little more sleep than I usually did. After many months, I noticed that I was exhausted by 9:30 pm. I also noticed that no matter what I did I was waking up at 5:00 am, rather than continually fighting my body's own nature, I decided to work with it. Making this little adjustment has relieved me of a great deal of stress. I began to see the advance of my health again. While fighting against nature and trying to hold onto old patterns, I felt a significant decline in my health and I battled an ongoing sinus issue that just wouldn't stop. Even with my expertise in health using herbs and diet and attempted lifestyle changes, I pondered where else it could be coming from. The core I believe was a simple lack of rest.

During this season as I adjusted to this new schedule, I felt more rested and alerted when I awoke and didn't feel as groggy. I also felt more peaceful about going to bed in the evening. I didn't feel quite so rushed and stressed in the morning as I woke the children for their day. Making subtle changes that reflect your body's unique need for rest, is one of the first areas you should address with regards to your health and the health of your family. It is a losing battle to continually fight against your body's own natural needs in the unique season you find yourself in at any given time in your life.

Being flexible as your life seasons change can make the greatest difference in your mental, physical and spiritual

Authentic Health

health. As we have moved our family back to the East Coast, we now have totally different schedules than we ever had before. Because Dad now gets home late, I allow the children to stay up later and to sleep in again. (I had never allowed sleeping in until this season of our family's life). But in order for my little ones to get enough rest, they need the latitude to sleep when they are tired and not be forced to be woken up before they are ready. I noticed a dramatic difference in their health while in school. They rarely got enough rest and I attribute the lowered immune system to the chronic lack of sleep. Even with early bedtimes, that pre-sunrise waking definitely took a toll on their health.

Let's make a pie

A healthy life is much like making a pie. You may think of all the pieces of the pie as a different value, but in order to have the more perfect and more delicious pie, all the ingredients must be present. Each ingredient comes together and synergizes to create the enjoyable dessert at the end of the baking process. If you think of life as a pie, you might divide it into seven categories. Here are some suggestions:

Authentic Health

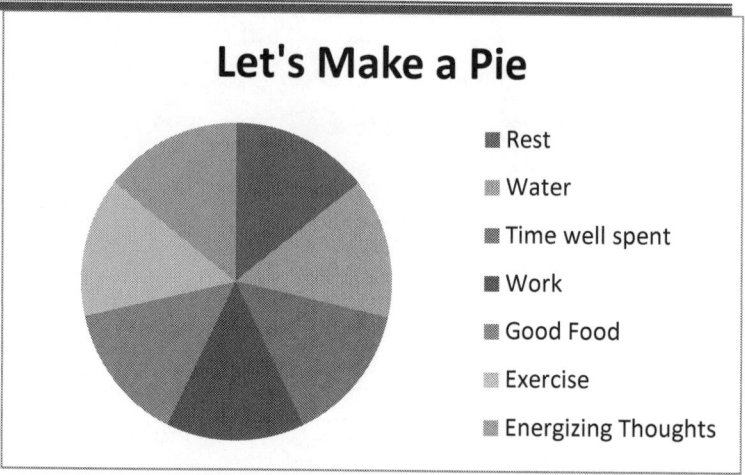

Healthy scheduling of commitments with the outside community relationships and many other areas could have been included. You alone can decide which areas should remain a part of your life's pie. But, I encourage you to realize that there is only so much you can be involved in at any given time. You can also not give yourself to your passions with so many distractions and do well with the things that matter most to you. When you try to stuff more than is reasonable into your pie plate, you sacrifice not only the appearance of your pie, but also the flavor of the individual pieces. Therefore, the first thing to recover and reclaim is your day.

When recovering your health becomes priority you will begin to be able to establish strategy to restore order to your day consistently, you can begin to develop new strategies for each season of your life and family that will allow for growth, as well as health in that area.

Authentic Health

PIE PIECE #1

Did you get enough rest today?

Rest is the first key. Getting sufficient rest is probably the essential key factor to health as without rest your body cannot heal. Contrary to popular misinformation, some people actually need 9 to 11 hours of sleep daily. Without rest they have greater general health loss and weight gain.

Children especially need 11 to 12 hours of sleep daily. I contribute the lack of sleep to the rising population of children labeled ADD and ADHD. The current model of children being dropped at daycare at 6:00 am and picked up at 6:00 pm to have an hour to eat dinner with their parents and then be bathed and put in bed, has not only contributed to the demise of the modern family, but also to the demise of the health of American children, the rise in childhood obesity, and the rise in medication use for children for behavioral disorders.

In my children, I have noticed a definite pattern of health improvement, or loss, when they are deprived consistently of healthy sleep patterns for their age group or body type. Smaller toddlers need a minimum of 9 to 11 hours daily. Without it they will begin to manifest colds and sickness. Their immune system will begin to drop, parasites will be easily acquired, and their body will not recover quickly from colds or flu. Their body's need to heal will become more and more obvious. This rest time gives them opportunity to do that healing.

PIE PIECE #2

Did you get enough water today?

The next area to address from a health perspective is water intake. Your body requires half of its body weight in ounces. For example, if you weigh 140 pounds you require 70 ounces per day to just meet minimum body requirements. Without it your body systems begin to function poorly. Your body's pH will shift and then your nutrient absorption will be impeded. Your glandular functions will slow. Your metabolism will shift. Your body will begin to gain weight and retain water. Your liver and kidneys will begin to function poorly and not purify blood completely, and your blood will actually become thicker than it should be. (This accounts for the rise in elderly of a medical need for "blood thinners" as the chronic lack of water intake is insufficient to maintain healthy blood.)

We know that we are thirsty in the summer when it's hot, but did you know that you need even more water in the winter, because you lose so much water to respiration and breathing? The important thing to remember is that you need to meet the goal. Without the necessary amount of water, essential body systems will suffer. In fact math skills decline, memory loss and headaches can occur when you are dehydrated.

PERCENTAGE OF WATER MAKE UP OF BODY TISSUES

Teeth	10%
Lungs	80%
Bones	13%
Brain	80%
Cartilage	55%
Plasma	90%
Bile	86%

Your body requires large amounts of water to function at its peak. Water enables the body to lubricate joints; carry nutrients to cells in the body; and carry waste materials out of the body. Water also enables the body to dilute high sugar levels which result from high carbohydrate intake or heavy sugar consumption. As the cells are filled with water, water helps them have shape weight and mass and to absorb and transport vital daily as well as repairative nutrients to the cells and other tissues, to

Authentic Health

bring daily health, as well as, healing. With limited hydration the tissue becomes dense and hardened, just like a dehydrated mushroom, unpleasant to look at, shriveled and lifeless.

Roles of Water

The following list shows some of the roles of water in the human body:

- Water transports nutrition and waste in and out of the cell
- Water helps extract vitamins, minerals, protein, and carbohydrates from foods and deliver it to the rest of the body
- Water removes harmful substances that could cause cellular death: carbon monoxide, nitrogen, ammonia and many others
- Without water you would have no digestive juices or enzymes to break down food
- Without water you would have no saliva
- Without water your eyes would be dry
- Water lubricates the joints and other tissues
- Without water your bones grate against one another
- Without water your organs would actually stick together
- Water also helps maintain internal temperature
- Without water we could not perspire

Authentic Health

Did you know these facts about water?

- 75 % of Americans are chronically dehydrated
- 37% of Americans mistake the thirst sensation, which is weak for the hunger sensation triggering them to begin eating instead of drinking
- mild dehydration can slow the metabolism by 3%
- drinking just one glass of water can shut down the "midnight munchies"
- lack of water is the number one trigger for daytime fatigue
- 8 to 10 glasses of water can ease back and joint pain in 80% of sufferers
- when you dropped just 2% in the body's necessary hydration you will likely experience fuzzy, short-term memory; and difficulty with basic mathematics; and difficulty focusing on printed work or computer media.
- Just by drinking five glasses of water daily you will decrease the risk of colon cancer by 45%; reduced risk of breast cancer by 79%; and 50% less likely to develop bladder cancer.

Clean and Clear

It is also important to drink pure, clean water. Water should be purified by reverse osmosis which works like the throat of a seagull. Seagulls drink salt water which flows through the membrane in the back of your throat which allows only the water to pass through the wall,

Authentic Health

they then spit out the salt. On the market today there are several brands which are actually R.O. purified. (Dasani and Aquafina to name a few.) They are required to put on their label the method of purification. Read your labels to be sure.

You may be asking what about distilled, isn't that purified? Yes, it is purified, but it is also a leaching water. Which means it will leach minerals from your system, thereby, de-mineralizing or aging or de-energizing you.

To read more about water read the book <u>Your Body's Many Cries For Water</u> by F. Batmanghelidj, M.D.

Does the temperature of the water matter?

Studies show that water can improve the speed of your weight loss: here's how!

Hot water, like the heat of hot tea, causes the body to begin to detoxify. Stored toxins slow the metabolism. When you flood the body with hot water, this causes the muscular action in the stomach, liver and intestine which squeezes and releases toxins. This moves toxins out of the bowel, liver, lymph system, and out of the body.

Lukewarm water suppresses appetite. When you include chlorophyll in a quart water, you will tend to drink more. Since the body takes in more water the vagus nerve turns off the hunger mechanism. Hunger pains diminish and you tend not to overeat. Water is also more quickly

Authentic Health

absorbed in extreme temperatures. This helps stabilize blood sugar, which will stop food cravings as well. Water temperatures effect the body's ability to cleanse, absorb and process bodily functions.

Lukewarm and hot have more healthful benefits. Cold water gives your body an entirely different effect. It causes your metabolism to speed up as much as 3% and a 10 minute time period. Why does this happen? The body has to work harder to warm the water so they can be absorbed and used by all of your cells. This thermogenic process utilizes large quantities of energy. Your body will then use its reserve tanks of stored back to release this energy.

In general the best temperature is lukewarm or room temperature water. If you are trying to elicit a cleanse hot water would be best. Cold water has limited benefits, though it can be refreshing on a hot day.

Other benefits from water:

Speed of Body Response & Effect

- 30 minutes: mental clarity increases by 20%
- That night: late-night hunger pangs disappear
- 24 hours: energy levels increase by 89%
- 72 hours: Blue or dark moods lift and sleep improves

Authentic Health

- four days: exercise endurance increases
- one week: chronic back pain subsides
- two weeks: joint pain eases
- three weeks : peptic ulcers begin to heal

Water wisdom:

The key to health with anything is consistency. Things done daily with determination will amass great long term gains. Practice starting the day with 8 ounces of hot lemon water. (Lemon causes the bile ducts to cleanse and strengthens the liver as well as improves digestion.) Practice alternating hot lemon water and icy water throughout the day (for weight loss benefits).

Drink lukewarm water 15 minutes before meals and snacks.

If weight loss is your goal, statistics show that by practicing these keys to water wisdom you can lose 31 pounds per year because you will consume 104 calories less daily as a result of drinking water.

All of the negative impacts which have been mentioned can be eliminated and avoided by simply having a glass of water.

Authentic Health

PIE PIECE #3---Healthy Food Intake

First, ask yourself how closely does the food resemble its' original state. For example, Apple versus Apple sauce; freshly made vegetable soup versus canned vegetable soup; and finally, venison or a store bought chicken. These are examples of foods from that are less processed, but what are some examples of foods that are not foods at all? Pop tarts, corn syrup, margarine, Cheez whiz, Campbell's soup. These examples are "non-foods". These should be avoided as they are or contain toxic ingredients, or highly allergenic ingredients.

When you are considering what to eat this week, start with a menu planner. With a visual plan you can easily see excessive grain intakes; you can see if you are lacking in vegetable or fruit intake and can see if you are even getting fats.

The chart does not have to be fancy just a simple table style chart. Four columns wide and eight columns down. One square for each meal of the week: breakfast lunch and dinner -- seven of each.

You can simply thematically choose your meals such as, using the meat as your foundation: Monday: poultry, Tuesday: meatless, Wednesday: beef, Thursday: wild game, Friday: fish, Saturday: leftovers, and Sunday: pot roast. Or, you could do a theme like Monday: stir Fry, Tuesday: stew, Wednesday: soup, Thursday: Mexican, Friday: Italian, Saturday: crock pot, and Sunday: leftovers

Authentic Health

A sample chart is pictured below:

Day	Brkfst	Lunch	Dinner
Mon			
Tues			
Wed			
Thur			
Fri			
Sat			
Sun			

However, you choose to organize your mind in food prep, a plan always saves you money and directs your thinking. Most importantly, the plan helps you rotate your foods. Food rotation helps you prevent reactions to food you are eating because it lessens the chance of creating an allergenic response to foods that are eaten too frequently.

Authentic Health

In spending a little time planning, you can help improve your health just by creating more variety in your daily diet. Also, your palette will never be bored. With a simple plan already designed by the week, you can make an appealing menu plan that will accomplish many nutritional goals. You can, at a glance, see that you will be meeting your daily vegetable and fruit goals, as well as being able to see if you are getting all that you planned to accomplish in your other nutritional areas like protein consumption, and grain rotation, etc. Most people are unfamiliar with grain rotation. However, grains are one of the primary allergenic factors in our diet and by simply watching frequency of consumption, a diet of moderation and few allergic responses can be achieved. This simple chart can help achieve a better more diverse diet.

Chapter 2: Going from Here to There

This Chapter will help you:

- ✓ Understand Basic Strategies for Health
- ✓ How to's of Planning your Strategy
- ✓ Achieving Your Goals- Begin with the End in Mind

Having a Strategy is Half the Battle!

Where do you want to go? Many people know they do not want to enjoy the poor health they have been experiencing, but have no idea where to begin.

The following are steps to reach your goals.

First, eat what God made. Eat it as close to how God made food as possible. The more raw uncooked or lightly cooked foods you eat the better your health will be.

Secondly, pray frequently. Release worry. Worry is an unproductive emotion the more energy you release into it the less solutions are produced. Studies have actually shown that prayer lowers the cortisol levels in the body. Cortisol is released by the adrenal glands when the body is under stress. When high levels of cortisol flood the blood, belly fat is produced. In order to avoid weight gain

Authentic Health

due to stress, it is important to understand this connection. Something as simple and freeing as prayer can eliminate a toxin with a negative impact on your body. Why not try prayer instead of worry in the future?

Third, remember rest is the key. A minimum of eight hours daily as a regular rule is needed by the body in order to maintain health. During times when this is not possible power naps can be used as a way to increase the percent of waking hours. Increasing effectiveness of the hours you are awake even while actually sleeping fewer hours. This has been a practice in the orient for centuries, as well as other cultures worldwide.

The fourth key is to focus on one front at a time. Don't try to fix everything at once. Just as housework goes better when you finish one task before beginning another; your body will also benefit from this approach. Chuck Pierce once said, "that every victory is to make you stronger for the next battle..."; so it is in life and health.

The fifth keys is taking your supplements consistently, nothing works unless you take it. People ask how long and how much will I take. Taking supplements for three months +1 month for every year a symptom has existed will generally correct the problem you have been experiencing. For example, if you have had low blood sugar or hypoglycemia for five years you will take supplements to repair the adrenals for 3+5 months a total of eight months. You will continue taking your supplements over the 8 months will repair the adrenals lands. How much should I take? Many people ask how much of a supplements are necessary to correct the problem? It takes 8 to 10 times the nutrition to repair

Authentic Health

and heal as it does to maintain. Initially you will be taking a larger quantity during the first three months than you will take the following months. The fourth and following months will be maintenance doses. This is generally the dose recommended on the bottle.

The sixth key is water. Remember half the body weight in ounces daily. Water is the key to cleansing at the cellular level. Without water and supplements repair and all else ceases.

The seventh key is to spend time in the sun daily. Daily exposure to the sun is essential to health. Even during the winter months getting some sun exposure is critical. 20 minutes daily in sunlight will make a huge difference in your immune system and emotional state. A brisk walk daily in the sun would go a long way to improving general health. If you live in an area of the country that this is impossible, then try to expose yourself to an infrared light or full spectrum bulb. These can be purchased in the lighting section of any home store. Full spectrum will fight winter blues or SAD (seasonal affected disorder) by stimulating the pineal gland. The infrared will also aid the pineal gland while also stimulating vitamin D production in the liver. An infrared sauna benefits the immune system; helps eliminate joint pain; increases strength and cardiovascular health; and much more. Infrared light, which is contained in sun light, helps the body maintain balance in physical and emotional health, as well as, benefits those who suffer with depression.

While these guidelines are extremely basic they are always essential to getting you to where you are going.

Authentic Health

Begin now to implement these seven basic steps to begin your approach to authentic health.

Plan a strategy for success

Strategy is essential to the success of your health journey. Without a map, most people never arrive at their destination. So first begin with a journal where you list each of your major health complaints. List the symptoms and severity of each issue you wish to address.

Number these symptoms from the newest to the oldest. This will enable you to place expectation to which symptoms will disappear first. The body will always heal in reverse order of how the symptoms have appeared. This means that if you have been experiencing arthritis symptoms for the last year, but prior to that had had digestive issues for many years, you can expect the arthritis to disappear before the digestive complaints will be alleviated entirely. This is due to the fact that the digestive issues were actually the original cause of the arthritis. The arthritis was simply a symptom of the original digestive problems. By addressing the digestive complaints specifically; you will actually alleviate the arthritis as well.

Once you have your list in front of you, you'll wish to use this book as a guide to determining your strategy. The strategy will include dietary changes, greater water intake, specific food strategies, and specific supplements strategies are, as well as, homeopathic remedies which will together speed your progress in achieving authentic health.

Authentic Health

What are your goals? Begin with these in mind

What would you like to accomplish? Do you simply want to be rid of symptoms? Or do you want to be revitalized; have more energy on moment to moment basis? The greater responsibility you take on everyday decisions about your health will allow you to choose the speed and level of success you experience.

I suggest you invest time in visualizing your ultimate goal. This goal may include personal goals or family goals. Visualize the details of what your goal looks like. Do you see yourself to enjoy greater physical activity, more mental prowess, greater levels of fitness, or just less sick days? Once you have visualized your destination it is time to begin your journey.

Chapter 3: Living High or on a Higher Conscious

This Chapter will help you:

- ✓ Learn to live at a higher frequency
- ✓ Take every thought captive
- ✓ Eat to live

The High Life: Your higher calling

As a parent we should seek not only to display the best example of how to live a rich life for our children, but also how to walk through life at a higher level of consciousness or awareness of the consequences of our actions and our thoughts. This should be in all areas of our life: moral, social, spiritual, educational, and even healthy lifestyle.

Your good example could be the prevention that allows your sons and daughters to outlive the current scientific predictions. Currently life expectancy is only 55 for the upcoming generation. For the first time in history the parents are expected to outlive their children. These statistics are based on health and disease trends which are only expected to rise, due to the epidemic of obesity and diabetes. Sadly, both of these conditions stem from dietary habits that can be controlled. We are the fattest nation on the planet and evidently the most foolish. It is certainly not a lack of availability of good foods. But instead a very poor set of repeated choices. Our children learn from us habits which ultimately are as deadly as taking illicit drugs.

The first important key to teach and live is to eat "live food." As much as possible, food should be eaten as it is found in nature. For example, eat an apple, instead of eating apple sauce. A salad should be eaten more often than a cooked vegetable. Enzyme value is lost in the heating process; the best choice is to eat raw uncooked foods as much as possible.

Next, eat with the seasons. Think how God sends different fruits in different seasons. Since God does nothing accidentally or out of season, it is best to eat as seasonal foods arrive naturally. For example, woody stemmed vegetables or cold weather crops, like potatoes, celery, carrots, broccoli, or cabbage are more abundant and nourishing in the winter. These would be examples of foods that should be consumed in abundance in the winter and colder seasons. These foods benefit the body by allowing it to store energy and produce heat or literal warmth. This warmth is needed to maintain life, especially during winter months. These foods also contain natural antidepressant qualities. Such as tryptophan and tyrosine which both naturally counter depressive moods.

Likewise, hot weather crops like watermelon, cucumbers and peaches have a cooling effect on the body and therefore should be eaten during hot seasons in order to manage body temperature more appropriately. Think of those hot summer months when a piece of watermelon tastes just right, quenching thirst and restoring blood sugar. It is refreshing and satisfying.

Beverages should also be consumed in temperatures appropriate to the need of the body. If you are running a fever that will not break, drink hot warming teas, like ginger or peppermint teas. These teas will activate the digestive system and stimulate the breaking of the fever, while soothing the body and keeping it hydrated.

Eat To Live

Another key to teach and live is the concept of balance in eating. The old teaching I remember that identified a balanced meal was centered around a square meal. This doctrine by no means denoted healthy eating, and as the current evidence proves Americans have by no means acquired the greater level of health that was promised.

Nor will history remember the current model as a health building pattern for eating. I believe that eating the quantity of carbohydrates that the "pyramid" model suggests will only manifest a "pyramid" figure, or a bottom heavy body. We see this appearing throughout our society as wide spread obesity has now over taken such a significant portion of the population. A problem with the pyramid model is the excessive quantity of carbohydrates this model suggested to eat. This heavy carbohydrate consumption coupled with a lifestyle without significant physical activity to burn these energy storing foods has created the image we now see him walking through the aisles of Wal-Mart and frequenting all you-can-eat buffets.

Another food model which is taught by Covert Bailey author of <u>Fit or Fat</u> is the circle. He suggests that it is best to eat within the circle. Anything that is in its natural, God-appearing state is near the center of the circle. This would include foods like seeds, nuts, fresh fruits and vegetables, cold pressed oils, and those meats that run until they are killed. For example, fish, bison, venison, goat, sheep and free range poultry would all fit the model of running meat sources. While pork, sea scavengers, and cattle are slow moving and consequently less healthy themselves. This makes their food value of a lesser quality than the other running food sources.

In fact, these foods, because of modern feeding practices, are generally unhealthy because of concentrated elements of the same foods. These create allergens or heavy sensitivities to both the animal and those ingesting the animals. For example, corn is a major feed for many of these animals. Corn has become a highly reactive food in the American diet. It is only logical that when a culture consumes large quantities of a single ingredient that it will become reactive or allergic to this ingredient. Corn syrup and corn derivatives are found in innumerable

Authentic Health

foods these days. Americans consume large quantities of these products daily. Couple this with the large quantity of corn which was spent originally to the animals to fatten them for market sale and we now have young people who are so sensitive to corn that they manifest behavioral problems, learning disabilities, and blood sugar imbalances as a result of continual consumption of corn and corn derived products.

Conversely, according to the circle model, the more altered the form of the food the less viable it is to the body. A tangible example of this is seen when you compare modern cereal to oatmeal. The cereal lacks so much nutrition that vitamins must be added back. In the foods' lack of satisfaction to the body, the body will eat more than is necessary because it is simply not satisfied.

Test this fact by trying to eat as many bowls of oatmeal (rolled oats) as you would of cereal. If you must use a boxed source for cold cereal I highly recommend the Kashi brand (which combines 7 ancient grains) or oat or spelt (which is an ancient relative of modern wheat that has less allergic response and provides a greater quanitiy of protein) flakes. You can enhance a bowl of whole grain flakes by adding dates, pecans or other nuts or dried fruits. Avoid corn flakes or corn products of any kind. Corn is used as a fattener. It is a fattener to the human body, just as it is for the cow going to market. You will notice that rarely do you eat more than a single bowl of higher-quality whole grain cereals. This is because the body's natural hunger mechanism is disabled when the body is satisfied.

Authentic Health

If you have problems getting through the day without snacking and are tempted to snack on unwholesome foods, try eating almonds. It takes around 9 to 11 almonds to stop the hunger mechanism by releasing lectins. This need to munch, is triggered by low levels of good fats in the body as well as low-level of quality protein. Almonds being a higher fat and high protein food are the perfect solution. Also, increase your healthy essential fats by taking krill oil, flax seed oil, or super Omega Fish oils. These will give you the needed calories which your body is craving in order to curb the desire for junky, fatty foods. Somewhere between four and six capsules a day of Super Omegas is all that is necessary to get the body loaded with high quality beneficial fats and free of these junky addictions. A tablespoon daily of Flax oil will accomplish the same.

Chapter 4:
The Vital Factor: Sleep

This chapter will help you:

- ✓ how to boost creativity
- ✓ improving weight loss
- ✓ lowering stress

Understanding this critical element will save your life:

Get enough sleep. At least eight hours is best, but power napping can be important too. Proper sleep allows the body to regenerate and heal. Without sleep our adrenals and immune system will begin to fail. When this happens overall health suffers. The body is no longer able to heal and repair the vital systems nor is it able to ward off attacks.

Even as I write this I have fallen victim to my own poor habits. After attending two births in the same night, and after 10 days I still do not feel I have recovered the time I lost in that one amazing night. Sleeping less than eight hours in two days, I am still recovering from falling for my own good advice. My immune system dropped, a cold set in, and now I must recover the sleep I missed a week and a half ago. No one is exempt from the requirements of good rest; sleep is a requirement for every healthy human body.

Authentic Health

The Power of the Power Nap

A "Power Nap" is a 20 to 30 minute nap in mid-day. This small break in the day can be a powerful solution to the sleep deprivation Americans struggle through. Power napping actually replaces missed sleep as well as boosting wakefulness. It also has the following benefits:

- boosting creativity
- raise motivation for physical activity
- increase cognitive ability
- improve heart function
- improve memory, alertness and productivity
- lower stress levels

Power napping is not to be a replacement for traditional sleep patterns. As the body's healing rhythm occurs during the night in our REM sleeping mode. This mode is not reached until we have been sleeping for 90 minutes or more. Power napping does not allow the body the benefit of REM: sorting through emotions, memories, and getting rid of stress.

Again, sleep is about balance between the repairative sleep: REM sleep mode and the power nap booster, which boost mental abilities and other processes.

We understand and acknowledge the necessity of proper sleep for infants, toddlers, and children. But somehow, we think we are free of bodily constraints like sleep after we hit our teen years. It all eventually catches up with us as adults. If we have not practiced good sleep habits throughout life, napping will not solve our problems.

Authentic Health

Poor sleep habits are inevitably connected with low immune systems, ADD, depression, mental fuzziness, chronic sickness, poor academic scores, high levels of stress, and weight gain.

The Results

When our body lacks critical sleep hours, we literally require greater quantities of calories just to maintain everyday activities. This accounts for the American habit of snacking constantly throughout the day. Imagine a young child's day in America. It begins by being awakened at 5:30am to be at daycare at 6:00am. He will not see the parents again until six at night, returning home to eat a quick fast food meal before bathing and being sent to bed. Also start the pattern again the next day. Couple this with a pop tart breakfast, "Lunchable" lunch, and McDonald's for dinner, and you have the makings for an American disaster. In a few years, this child is facing such situations as food allergies, poor academic scores, ADD., ADHD behavior, and obesity. Not to mention he is now a candidate for diabetes in later life, as well as, premature death.

Americans do however have other choices, but it may require parents making a different decision than the decisions that were made for them. Scaling down lifestyles or creating opportunities so that mothers can work from home.

For now, start where you are. Begin to commit to go to bed before 11:00pm or 10:00pm or whatever time tends to be where you push yourself to, and then past. I once committed to going to bed before midnight for an entire

Authentic Health

year, that year I experienced no sickness whatsoever. Unfortunately, I did not continue this practice. Following that year, I began experiencing minor sicknesses again, always connected to a period of 3 to 4 days without sufficient sleep. As with all human's, no one can violate the rule of rest. This essential factor keeps the body healing, recovering and clear headed.

Chapter 5: How to make A Healthy Baby

This chapter will help you obtain the following goals:

- ✓ Achieving Pregnancy
- ✓ Enjoying a healthy pregnancy
- ✓ Having a healthy birth

It all starts with YOU!

A healthy baby is the product of a healthy mom. An apple tree can only produce apples. Likewise your body can only pass on what it has to offer. The gene pool is affected by the body's health at the time of conception. If there is a fertility struggle the body is likely not in the best form to carry a child to full term and produce a healthy product.

If your body is having fertility issues, it is likely that your body needs to cleanse, become more alkaline as well as rebuild the glandular network. Following these protocols will improve the likelihood of conception.

Authentic Health

The following protocol is a good place to begin:

- bowel cleansing
- pH balancing (alkalizing system)
- improve hormone function
- improve thyroid function
- improve blood sugar levels

Bowels should function three times daily. Yes, I said three eliminations daily. If you are not having three eliminations daily, you are not functioning at peak. Try using Bowel Detox, two capsules twice daily. If you have chronically experienced constipation, this would be anything less than twice daily, you should consider using a Taio He cleanse for a 10 to 15 day period to unblock the bowels before attempting to do maintenance. Bowel Detox would function as a maintenance protocol only. Bowel toxicity can cause the body to be over acid and actually kill sperm as it enters the womb. Therefore, this is the first place to begin.

pH balance is the next critical element in the fertility process. The body's pH can be a direct result of the body's inability to eliminate waste. The first step to pH balancing is bowel cleansing as we just mentioned. The next critical steps involve proper digestion and calcium uptake. A pH protocol is included in the appendix.

The next step is to get critical glandular functions in order. If you have had a past of irregular cycles, try using Menstrual Reg this formula will begin to normalize the glandular function. If you have experienced cramping and heavy cycles, Cramp Relief is the formula that will balance your glandular system. If there has been a long history of many reproductive irregularities, Female

Authentic Health

Comfort would be indicated. If your body does not have interest in the romance of marriage, your testosterone levels are likely low. Try using Maca to improve and balance testosterone levels. Maca is a beneficial supplement for both men and women, as it is a testosterone balancer and increases the libido in both men and women.

Low thyroid levels can also contribute greatly to infertility. Statistically, mothers who have low functioning thyroid's are more likely to produce a child with a low IQ or lower level intelligence or even mental retardation. Therefore, it is important to protect and nourish your thyroid before and during the pregnancy. As iodine is the critical nutritional element for the thyroid function and it is also a critical element in the function of the immune system. Black walnut and thyroid activator are two effective formulas for promoting and improving thyroid function and increasing iodine levels.

The last area of concern is the blood sugar levels. High or low blood sugar levels can greatly affect the body's ability to conceive and carry. It is common that the body will need to have support during pregnancy, as if it is a diabetic and sugar levels fluctuate. Try using Target P 14 to regulate the body's blood sugar. Blood sugar levels shift greatly depending on the levels and quantity of fiber and good fats. It is important that the body maintain high levels of good fats. These essential fatty acids are found in foods like Flax seed oil or Super Omega's or Krill oil. Using these supplements prior to and during pregnancy as well as during nursing, will greatly improve the health of the pregnancy, as well as benefit the mom, while nursing. Good quantities of fat are essential for

Authentic Health

brain development for the unborn child as well as the child who has already arrived. So, do not neglect using essential fatty acids.

Fiber is the other essential element to blood sugar balancing. Fiber helps our bodies feel full, as well as to eliminate toxins from the bowel. Adequate amounts of fiber will keep bowel function healthy. Good sources of fiber are found in fruits and vegetables not in bread or cereals. The best thing during pregnancy and after pregnancy is to eat a large salad each day. Couple this with several servings of fruits throughout the day and your body should not lack of fiber.

Once these areas are met, pregnancy is much easier to achieve. These areas are extremely important not just in the achievement of pregnancy but also in the maintenance of pregnancy. A simple smoothie daily that includes several key ingredients could make all the difference of a successful healthy pregnancy.

A simple fruit smoothie with tablespoon of Flaxseed oil and a teaspoon of Natures Three, along with a scoop of Coral Calcium and Ultimate Greenzone would maintain great basic nutrition, as well as great preparation for delivery. Following the birth this smoothie is also be a great way to maintain general nutrition for mom and baby. And the smoothie will help baby sleep through the night as well.

Chapter 6: Healthy Beginnings: Pregnancy, Birth & Beyond

In this chapter you will:

✓ Consider the impact of beliefs on your birth outcome
✓ Be exposed to birth options you have not considered
✓ Have the freedom to choose where you must be

Birthing is a sacred event

The birthing process is not only very important, private and sacred, but also very critical to the formative health and emotional development of your baby. According to many, the birthing process is where the baby's psyche attaches itself to one of seven foundational fears. You can read more about this in Karol Truman's <u>Feelings Buried Alive Never Die</u>.

In this book she asks the reader to consider that for many of us our fathers may not have been allowed to be present at your birth. Until the mid 1970's fathers were expected to be in the waiting room, awaiting the heroic doctor's arrival to announce as if he were Gabriel himself that the child has been born. The child is aware of the presences at his birth, particularly those of his parents. Their absence is likewise noticed. A sense of emotional abandonment can set in at an early age, as well as, a lack of bonding, thereby affecting the relationship the rest of the child's life.

The true hero in the picture is the mother, not the doctor. She did all the real work; he just showed up to collect the insurance fees. I may sound cynical, but I have heard too many horror stories of what "the butcher" did to the trusting mother's body while "doing his job." My husband delivered my last four babies with me. He treated my body with the same respect as in the marriage bed. He treated me as if it were his own body. I realize that this is an extreme position for many families and that not every father or mother feels equipped to birth at home unattended by a medical practitioner. For us, after five other healthy deliveries and much training from four different midwives, we felt equipped and prepared for this most empowering experience. (Read the birth stories at the end of the book.)

There is always the tradition of women being helped by other women, as in many social cultures where midwives attend female family members. Again the body is shown respect, the woman is empowered and healthier families are bound closer and closer together. The total dependence on people, not technology, is incredibly honoring to the human being. Birth is one of the oldest human experiences. Birth has occurred naturally without interventions, drugs or episiotomies since the time of the Garden of Eden.

Many people have not considered that this traditional method of birth is still available to them. And therefore do not consider this option. I was thankfully not one of those people. Where this internal information came

Authentic Health

from I do not know, but it has always been my desire to have my children at home.

When I announced to my mother that I was expecting my first child, she too knew that this was the way it would be for me. She told me that she had read an article about a nearby midwife and that perhaps I should find out who that article was written about. My mother had never considered home birthing herself, having had all of her children, in a hospital, in stirrups with an epidural and my father in the waiting room for all but the last of us.

I have now had all nine of my children at my own home, enjoyed the comfort of a soothing woman's voice with my first five and the strength of my husband's calm voice during the final four "intimate" births. At the most climatic moments of my life as a new life birthed from me, I have enjoyed the welcoming, or homecoming, of my children into my home and enjoyed sleeping in my own bed, bathing in my own bath, and all the comforts that only home has. (I realize that this option is frightening to some people. However, given exposure to alternative or traditional birth options and the right tools and information, you will likely consider options beyond the fear driven medical model.) You must be where you must be to have your baby. You must be where you feel comfortable and cared for.

I remember my first midwife explaining that you would never consider moving a cow into the vet's office for her to have her calf. This made so much sense. I, like the cow, had no desire to be rushed somewhere other than my own bedroom. There is nothing like bringing life into the space you feel most restful in. There is also nothing like driving up to a house and remembering who was born there.

What if there are complications?

Some of you are asking, what if they're complications? In all honesty, you are more likely to have complications from a hospital delivery where all the germs are foreign to your system. In a setting which is not your natural ecological environment disease lingers in the literal air your child will breathe. Your birthing attendant is not concerned only for your care, but perhaps and likely for several other laboring women. His or her attention is not for you alone. Your personal well being is not of primary concern but rather that rules and policy be complied with. The pervading sense is that every bodily function is some type of emergency that must be treated or managed in some type of scientific laboratory and sterile environment.

The contrast of a midwife attended home delivery is striking. The attendant is there on a constant moment to moment basis for you and your baby. You and your spouse can function in unison and the midwife is there in a support role, listening to your needs and thoughts, and guiding you to a successful, empowering experience.

My midwives have always had nothing on their mind but me, my baby and our safety. A good midwife will know long before delivery if there are going to be problems and she will let you know if she suspects that alternative plans need to be arranged.

Authentic Health

There are so many procedures which are now standardized in hospital deliveries that are basically barbaric. Episiotomies have no place during delivery or any other time. There is no reason to believe that your body cannot remove what was planted there. On occasion, there is tearing during delivery. However, good midwife can help prevent this with perineal massages and oil poultices. I have had no tearing during my nine labors. Only once did I have any type of birth trauma internally. This was because of my own impatience. I should have pushed a few more times, instead of the more forceful push that brought my Felicia into the world. I had what the midwife described as skid marks inside the birth canal.

Since that birth, I always use evening Primrose oil. I take two capsules daily as well as using it internally. It is best to insert the capsule at night. The body absorbs the little gel cap entirely. This softens and moisturizes the cervix and gives greater elasticity to that area of the body.

Another thing to guard is your mind. During pregnancy you should not sit anticipating problems. Be informed and prepared, yes. Know what to expect during labor and delivery. Yes, there is pain. But this is pain with a purpose, a beautiful purpose, whose name is life. Do not fear. Most women make their decisions based on fear. Fear of pain. Fear of complications. Fear of what others will think. It is only important what you and your husband believe. Your two opinions are the only ones that matter. You must have a sense of peace about your decision. With this sense of peace, you will have a successful and rewarding birth experience.

Authentic Health

I pray that you will consider the unconventional, but formerly most conventional approach to birth. Statistically, the safest place to be is in your own home. It is the most natural place to be. It is where all of our forefathers were born. It is where most if not all children belong. This is, I understand, a challenging thought to the general public who has not challenged themselves by thinking past what the media, and medical fear mongers have trained us to believe. Women have been disempowered for almost a century by the medical model of child birth. The disempowerment is so distinct that the American woman having a hospital birth has a one in three chance of delivering by C-section. The incidence of induction deliveries in the states is around 40%, meaning 4/10 women will be induced to begin their labors. And, one of two women birthing in hospital will have episiotomies. Each of these barbaric experiences is actually paid for by the family of the patient. The cost with each added service is extraordinary. And don't be fooled, you are paying even if you have insurance.

Basically, the odds of a wonderful, spiritual experience are greatly against the mother and baby. Complication creation is a large part of the hospital mind set. Go prepared for this attitude when you enter that paradigm.

But I must emphasize that the mother must be where she feels most secure. She should have a known plan written out, and especially if having a hospital birth, have a doula and husband or birth partner who will represent your pre-decided views when you are not able to speak for yourself. Do not allow the baby out of your sight following his arrival. Also consider the choices connected with vaccines, circumcision, vitamin K shots,

Authentic Health

etc. before you enter the hospital. Make sure the hospital remembers they are working for you and not you for them. Some hospitals are more open to some natural methods. It is important to ask questions of your hospital and your doctor before the delivery. Know what you are supposed to expect and make your desires known emphatically.

A midwife will be very aware that she is there to serve your needs and not hers. She will educate as well as bring wisdom, experience and knowledge to the event. Value, I believe, is the word, not monetary but spiritual. This value is brought to the most extraordinary experience of a lifetime. I am fortunate to have experienced this most empowering event not only once but nine times personally. This fact still amazes me. I have also been blessed to be an attendant at other births to bear witness to the miracle as an observer and encourager.

To ensure a healthy birth, it is important to remember that this event is just the turning of a chapter. The story actually began with a seed being planted. Hopefully, the seed has been planted in healthy soil, figuratively speaking. Begin by getting both parents as healthy as possible, balancing glands, like the thyroid, adrenal and of course reproductive glands.

Many times I counsel with couples who say they desperately want children but have little energy or interest in the very activity that produces a child, sex. I often ask, if you say you want a garden but don't want to plant seeds, I question your true desire to see flowers grow. It is critical to address the area of energy, vitality and libido before conception if possible as a healthier mom experiences a healthier lower risk pregnancy than an unhealthy mom. She will also recover faster and have more energy for the baby upon arrival.If the reproductive glands are off, libido may be low or vaginal dryness may be a problem. The ovulatory cycles may be irregular as well. The following protocols can be beneficial in bringing balance to the glandular system:

Pregnancy Boosters for the different Phases of Pregnancy

Maca: to balance the libido, thyroid and adrenal glands. This supplement can be beneficial to both parents

Damiana: is used to increase strength of egg and sperm. Again, this is beneficial to both parents

During Pregnancy

Liquid chlorophyll: taken several times daily helps alkalize the body. Helps achieve pregnancy and can be used throughout pregnancy to keep blood supply strong and helps prevent hemorrhaging.

Red raspberry: is used to strengthen the uterus, making labor and delivery and recovery more efficient. It is also great as a tummy tuck following, tightening the muscles of the abdomen wall

Ginger: is beneficial for those who suffer with nausea or morning sickness. Two capsules taken as needed, will greatly reduce these symptoms.

Authentic Health

I –X: an herbal iron supplement. Is used to improve the body's ability to circulate oxygen to the cells and reduce the risk of swelling and preeclampsia & toxemia. Keeps body from Anemia.

Skeletal Strength: Once conception has occurred it is important to take Skeletal Strength in order to boost calcium supplies and raise pain threshold in preparation for delivery.

Supplements for Special times in Pregnancy

LBS II. In order to keep the bowels working easily. This will help reduce the severity of inflammation which is ultimately the cause of constipation& hemorrhoids.

Varigone: If hemorrhoids or varicose veins are a problem, then take Varigone capsules and apply bear God cream topically to shrink and eliminate. This can be useful following pregnancy and following the birth. If you have a tendency to hemorrhoids, you should take

Evening Primrose oil should be used the month prior to the due date daily as a supplement and also used internally, as this will begin to both ripen the cervix as well as moisturize the tissue to prevent tearing,

During the delivery

When I go into labor I usually eat a hearty meal. Lots of protein and drink tons of chlorophyll water. I drink about half gallon or gallon during the course of the labor and following. This will lessen bleeding and decrease risk of hemorrhaging. This will also strengthen blood supply and boost milk production following the birth. Chlorophyll is a vital part of pregnancy, birth, and nursing.

If you are in a hospital setting, you may likely not be allowed to eat or drink. They will usually only give chipped ice for hydration, while simultaneously giving a saline or salt solution intravenously. This causes the body to become saturated with fluids and swell, making labor more difficult and blood pressure elevated. This creates more risk in the birth setting the longer you are there. Hospitals are always prepping for surgery. The risk of vomiting under anesthesia is the reason why food is denied. Yet a long labor requires much energy and nutrients, prepare for birth with a good healthy high protein meal.

I remember my births where I had eaten well before going into labor. These births went much better because my strength had substantial nutrition to fall back on. However, in middle of the night births, I was more fatigued following the birth and famished. Best to plan ahead and even have some meals prepared ahead in the freezer for following the birth.

Zinc supplementation is essential to prevent postpartum blues. Postpartum blues can be more involved than just the feeling of depression, you can actually lose appetite and all interest in food. This is due to the increased need for zinc during pregnancy and during nursing. Somewhere around 50 to 75 mg zinc daily is necessary to keep mom feeling sane. If you are a vegetarian or not a heavy meat consumer, you will have to make sure to take the additional zinc as the highest natural source is red meat. In fact, you would need 2 pounds of red meat daily or 2 gallons of lima beans to equate the necessary zinc in a day.

Homeopathy for pregnancy.

Arnica: This remedy is used for muscle aches from physical exertion and may also be used to treat shock. The remedy is also found to be very valuable in helping to recuperate from the childbirth process.
Belladonna: is used when women exhibit signs of nervousness, agitation and deliriousness. Other symptoms include flushing of the face, mucus membranes and skin which is hot to the touch.
Caulophyllum / Blue Cohosh: Used for strengthening uterine muscles which can help process of labor. This is also used for irregular contractions or weakening of the uterus during labor.
Cimicifuga: is used for spasmodic pains and may also be used for those who are intolerant of pain.
Pulsatilla: This is a common medicine for helping to to turn a breech baby late in pregnancy.
Staphysagria: If a caesarean or episiotomy becomes necessary, this is used to help the healing process and is given after surgery.
Sulphur: This helps to prevent tearing and stretching of tissues around the bladder and vaginal area.

Authentic Health

Following the birth

Eat a hearty meal and sleep as much as the endorphins will allow you. I always spend time taking pictures of baby and daddy and family with baby. Then I rest.

I know everyone says sleep when baby sleeps and they are right, though this is more difficult when there are other children in the house. Consider asking a grandparent or friend to take your other children at least the day following the birth when you will suddenly be aware of your need for sleep. Or have a doula stay with you to guard noise and help around the house a bit.

Be sure to have someone there who you know will guard you and buffer the rest of the household to allow time to recover and regenerate. Don't have a person there who though well meaning, brings stress with their very presence. This will not speed the healing process but rather inhibit and slow it.

In the days following birth you can expect to feel tired; chlorophyll will help regenerate and help bleeding end more quickly. If you are feeling any sort of emotional lows that might lead to post-partum blues, take Milk Thistle or Blessed Thistle. These will aid the liver in detoxification, as often the liver has been over taxed while cleansing both your blood and the baby's blood.

Authentic Health

Supplements for Post Birth Healing

Golden Salve: This also helps to speed up healing process via salve form. This is particularly beneficial to mother if there is any tearing, as it will aid in restoring the tissue and keeping infection from tissue while healing. It will also add soothing moisture to the torn tissue.
Varigone: This is helpful following a birth which have involved a lot of pushing and result in hemorrhoids. The Varigone Cream can be applied topically to the area and will take even severe bleeding hemorrhoids down in about three days. Taken internally should there be hemorrhoids during pregnancy will alleviate pain, discomfort and reduce the swelling.
Red Raspberry: This herb should be taken throughout pregnancy. However following pregnancy is extremely beneficial as it will help tighten to the uterus to return it to it's original size. It will also encourage milk production are nursing.
Zinc: is one of the most important supplements, you could take throughout pregnancy as well as postpartum nursing days. The body requires 3 to 4 times that of a person who is not pregnant or nursing. Therefore it is critical that one supplement with 2 to 3 tablets of zinc daily, in order to maintain healthy mental function and a healthy appetite. In order to acquire enough zinc to maintain healthy levels one would have to eat to 2 pounds of beef daily in order to just meet the needed requirement. 2 to 3 tablets is a small investment in balancing moods and keeping a healthy appetite during nursing.

Authentic Health

Homeopathics for Post-Partum

Arsenicum album: A woman who needs this remedy feels extremely insecure about her situation, wanting constant help and support. She can be extremely picky and controlling toward others-or seem very restless, yet exhausted and incapable. Women who need *Arsenicum* sometimes feel despair from insecurity, with thoughts that deeply frighten them.
Aurum metallicum: When this remedy is indicated, depression can be dark and despairing. The woman may feel worthless and see little point in life. Problems may be worse at night, or when weather is dark and days are short. Women troubled by depression in the past (not necessarily related to pregnancy) are often likely to respond to *Aurum*. Professional help could be necessary if depression is severe.
Calcarea carbonica: This remedy can be helpful to a woman who is overwhelmed by working too hard and taking on too much responsibility. Weakness and fatigue make her feel depressed. Anxiety, insomnia, and nightmares may develop. A person who needs this remedy often feels sluggish, cold, and easily tired by exercise.
Cimicifuga: This remedy is often useful when a woman is depressed for both emotional and hormonal reasons. She may feel "a dark cloud" has crept over her life and that everything is wrong. Extremely anxious and gloomy, she may start to think herself incapable of caring for the baby-or she may become excitable and talkative, saying and doing irrational things.
Ignatia: helps if mother feels tense, upset, or grief-stricken after childbirth. The grief may be for an actual loss (for instance, the baby may have health problems); but often occurs if the birth was difficult, and not as beautiful as she imagined. Defensiveness, hysterical behavior, sighing, sudden outbursts of tears or laughter, and insomnia are indicators.

Natrum muriaticum: This remedy can be helpful to a woman who feels sad and sensitive, and wants to be alone to cry. She may be brooding and withdrawn, anxious about her mothering abilities, or doubtful and discouraged about her relationship with the baby's father or other family members. Despite her sadness, she may seem angry or offended if anyone tries to console her. Women who need this remedy may also have headaches or palpitations when depressed.

Phosphorus: A woman who needs this remedy has an active imagination with tremendous fear-thinking of every possible danger or misfortune that might occur. She is very worried that she won't be able to cope if something happens, and terrified that harm might come to the baby. She often wants constant company and feels afraid to be alone. A woman who needs this remedy may also have a tendency toward easy bleeding and exhaustion, which may have added to her fear and nervousness.

Pulsatilla: This remedy is often indicated for women who are emotional, tearful, and sensitive in situations involving hormonal changes. The woman may feel extremely insecure and needy-wanting constant affection, reassurance, and nurturing. She is likely to feel worse when warm and in a stuffy rooms, improving after crying and from being out in open air.

Sepia: This remedy may be helpful to a mother who feels worn out and indifferent after childbirth, and does not want other people making demands or expecting anything of her. She may have trouble bonding with the baby, and may not even want to have it close to her. Most women who are in need of this remedy feel resentful and overburdened (though some only feel exhausted, irritable, and sad). A feeling that the pelvic floor is weak or that the uterus is sagging are other indications for *Sepia*.

Authentic Health

Fact Links:

With induction brings a 50% higher incidence of cesarean section.

With the 2007 rate at 31.8%, about one mother in three now gives birth by cesarean section, a record level for the United States. (http://www.childbirthconnection.org/article.asp?ck=10456)

There was an overall episiotomy incidence of 48%; obstetricians performed episiotomy in 54% (http://www.jabfm.org/cgi/content/full/18/1/8)

When considering traditional vs non-traditional (homebirth or intimate birth) you should be aware of real facts, not just inferences from your doctor.

Pregnant in America & The Business Of Being Born are both excellent material to view by DVD to become more educated about the true facts of American child birth.

Chapter 7: Birth Stories

Your birth reflects your state of mind:

- ✓ consider the physical
- ✓ consider the emotional
- ✓ consider the spiritual

Your Birth Reflects Your Prevailing Attitude

Fear of the unknown is particularly common with first pregnancy. That's why it's important to read and educate yourself as much as possible. Looking back I wished I had read more stories by women like myself. Reading other birth stories would have at least educated me to the heroic thinking, as well as, the experience of birth.

The Number One Son

Christian's pregnancy had been difficult at best. We had determined immediately that we would have our baby without a doctor and instead use the wisdom a midwife. The midwife care model is far superior to that of a doctor. An expectant mother gets not only caring support, but also empowering education about your body and the process of birth. Our first midwife was the perfect blend of all these things. She was a midwife of 24 years, a nurse and a nutritionist. She offered as much information as we could ask for. The birth of our first child was attended by this wonderfully wise and experienced woman, herself a mother of 2.

Unfortunately, my health during this time of my life was still in the early stages of recovery. My liver was so weak from many years of pharmaceutical drug therapy for allergies and ear, nose and throat problems, that at less than 5 months of pregnancy I was swollen and bloated. By the time I delivered I weighed 170 pounds and my blood pressure was elevated to a dangerous level. In fact, my midwife had intended to hospitalize me the day after our home visit following her consultation with a doctor concerning my situation. But her other February baby came due and this delayed the call for my admission into the hospital. This gave my body the necessary opportunity for the herbal program I went on to have time to manifest the need effect.

Following my midwife's final pre-birth visit, I felt very sad and discouraged because she had told me she was uncertain as to my strength to complete the birth in a home setting. After she left I recalled some information sheets which an herbal friend had given me months before that discussed pregnancy and herbal solutions. I began reading some notes on problems during pregnancy and noticed toxemia, preeclampsia and saw what I needed to do. As soon as I learned what to take to correct this problem, I began taking the I-X formula at a double dose, 4 three times daily. Within 2 days, the swelling had miraculously come out of my hands and feet. Sharing this information convinced the midwife that I would be okay to deliver at home.

Authentic Health

This birth was about 6 hours long, and very painful. The newness and fear of the unknown contributed greatly, not to mention the fear of motherhood itself. However, the birth went well, and I delivered my new baby, Christian. I recall feeling like a human water slide, as the last push thrust my new son out into the world. Strangely, as I complete this work he is sixteen and finishing the last few months of his home education. And will again be thrust into the world, like a cannon shot.

Following the birth, I continued using the I-X. Thanks to the use of I-X (an herbal iron supplement) which helps cleanse the liver and kidney, I was able to in 4 days to relieve my body of over 40 pounds of fluid. I also took Liquid Chlorophyll, and Liquid Calcium to help support my very weak body. During the most intense time of the birth, I remember being given Dong Quai to help strengthen me for the last of the birthing process. This helped to sustain me through the intense time. Christian's birth was the beginning of entering the unknown of parenthood. The intensity of labor was added to by the fact that this journey held so many unknowns. We had not planned to have a child this soon. But God knew it was time for us to get serious about our life, and Christian began that journey with us. And set us in motion to become who we were to be.

Following his birth, I noticed discomfort during intimacy. This was due to a little nick as my little boy's shoulders passed out of my body. I also had extreme vaginal dryness. I didn't know at the time that this dryness was very common during nursing. Once I learned this I began using Evening Primrose oil internally to soften and moisten that tissue and speed healing to that area. I also used a homeopathic of Cal. Sulph which aids tissues that are slow to heal. Within just two days of using that homeopathic the tissue had healed. I used it again following my second birth to find similar fast healing results.

Felicia Joy's Joyous entry...

My second birth, as unlike the first as the two children's personalities began on a Sunday morning early. Felicia's entire delivery was again six hours from the first contraction to the last. However, this birth lacked the fear, risk or concerns. Very much like Felicia, I had no fear of the unknown, no inhibitions, and thankfully nothing but joy surrounding her arrival. The unseen elements of the mother's emotions, expectations and the perhaps, well hidden, unseen secret fears can put a spin on a birth that is unexpected and potentially negatively affect the process of birth. Thankfully, with Felicia no fears or qualms surrounded her arrival. She was wholly accepted, planned and welcomed into our family. The birthing experience totally reflected the calm and determined reception.

My mother, and of course Steven were present along with the two midwives who attended. We chatted throughout the preamble to the actual intense time of labor, then as contractions would come I would stand stretch and breath. I got into the tub as the labor got more intense, but only stayed a few minutes as the intensity level jolted to a crescendo very quickly. Following my brief tub time, I had only a few brief minutes of pushing and our precious baby, Felicia Joy has shot into the world.

Authentic Health

I have never been known as a particularly patient person, and as the birth neared the end, I decided to give one final push, this would be the final push, as I did she shot out. Later I learned the folly of this type of determination. I actually had skid marks, like a strawberry from sliding into home plate, except on the interior tissue, from that last push. Calc Sulph had to heal that again. Unfortunately, this time I did not take it for a year, not remembering the former effectiveness until I was researching for another friend with similar problems. I later learned that Evening Primrose oil used internally for the final month of pregnancy along with 5-W formula would prevent this type of trauma from reoccurring. With that knowledge I never had any form of tearing again. Thank you, God for wisdom and knowledge for the daily journeys of motherhood, from start to finish.

The Premature Arrival

My next child's arrival was equally accepted and the birth like our life at the time, was a whirlwind. We had been living in an apartment in the back of our office far longer than the intended 6months of finding a new house where we had opened our first wellness center. We had expected 6 months or so to find a house in the area, but in reality we found the house after 2 years and 3 months, the space between my two girls. We moved in 1 week before Charity's 3 week pre-mature arrival.

I had insisted jokingly that I would not have this baby until all the curtains were hung. I had a friend over and hung the shower curtain, the last curtain in the house and immediately felt a twinge in my lower back. Less than 3 hours later, Charity had arrived. Her birth like our move went fast and was over before you had time to think. My water had broken while I was having contractions and I did not have the usual breaking of waters that was a single distinct event. I had delayed the call to the midwife. I was three weeks before due date so I didn't want to call with a false alarm. But by the time I realized that this was not a false alarm, it was an urgent call to come quickly.

Her birth was a late afternoon birth and Steven had not yet come home. Thanks to my sister-in-law, who went back to the office and told my husband to hurry because she too was coming to attend the birth and had gotten the call to hurry. He had not realized that his call was urgent and not just a call to come home, but a "GET HOME NOW" call.. These were the days before cell phones of pagers.

The final minutes of Charity's arrival were as follows:

20 minutes before arrival: midwife arrives

15 minutes before arrival my mother arrives (house had no working plumbing we discovered after closing, so much for home inspections)

10 minutes before arrival sister in law arrives with toilet paper

5 minutes before arrival Steven arrives

2 pushes later baby arrives. Charity is born.

I recall asking the midwife to break the water, because the pain had gotten so intense. She went to check my progress and informed me that the water sac was long gone and that what I was feeling was not the sac but the head. Two pushes and there was my beautiful baby girl, Charity. She had the signs of a slightly pre-mature baby: little peanut like nubs under her nipples, the ears had not quite rolled over at the top, and only a third of her foot print was visible.

Sometime when things seem early or out of time, they are indeed exactly on time. We had a friend who had been contemplating and even scheduled an abortion of her unborn baby for the following Monday. I had prayed that if my baby needed to come early to prevent this, that God would intervene. He did and the friend saw Charity on Saturday and canceled the appointment. The two girls have been playmates for their lifetime. God's hand pushed her out a little early so that she could save another. God is amazing.

The Southern Belle

My final Virginia birth, Linnea Charisse was another wonderful birth. This would be another Sunday afternoon delivery like Felicia. Throughout the pregnancy I had been obsessed by studying flowers and gardening. She is named after the national flower of Sweden and is derived from the name of the scientist who developed the study of botany. Because we thought she would be a boy, her name was given two days post delivery, being called simply baby until a name could come forth, for the non-male we had unexpectedly produced.

Her delivery started very calmly at 4:30 in the morning. But I had so much more I wanted to accomplish that day.

Authentic Health

I got busy on my tasks and stopped the labor by about 11:00am. The midwives left our home and said to call when labor started again. The house quieted down, Steven and I took a nap and then about 1:30 things picked up where they left off. Even now, I recall looking out the window on that breezy April afternoon to see all the two hundred tulips we had planted, the garden pond I had dug following Charity's birth and all the spring colors bursting forth. Shortly after, I forced her out. I say forced because, she had an unusual presentation. Charisse arrived face first. She did not crown, but had tipped her neck upwards and wrapped the cord like a beauty queen's sash across her shoulder, this pushed the neck in the air. Presenting her face first, not the usual crown first; this presentation was the reason for the delayed process of her birth.

Even though her birth was difficult from presentation perspective, there was only a short window of intensity. During the last minutes of the birth, I felt that I might tear, but thanks to the preparation of Evening Primrose and the 5 W, I had no tearing. This was amazing considering the presentation. Evening Primrose helps maintain elasticity of the tissue and softening of the cervix. Following birth is encourages healing and restoration. It definitely worked as there was no evidence of the trauma of her birth. Just the joy remained!!!

Authentic Health

Liberty's entrance

Our fifth child arrived along the trail of our next adventure. We were living in Pennsylvania at the time. We had to find a midwife there, because we did not have any connections to find one as in Virginia. However, unlike Virginia where midwifery was a misdemeanor, midwifery was a respected profession and actually advertised in the Yellow Pages. Without much difficulty a midwife was found to guide us through the delivery of our fifth child.

Her pregnancy was very uneventful outside of redoing and 11 room house. My labor began in the late afternoon while on a playground playing with my children. I headed home and began preparations for the delivery. Early that morning, I had sat in quiet time and began to read <u>The Encyclopedia of Country Living</u>. Strangely, the book opened to a page on what to do if you delivered your baby by yourself unattended, assisted. It included this action or what to do if the baby was a "noosling" meaning that the cord was wrapped around the baby's neck. I remember thinking that this would be the case with this baby. God was preparing us, for simultaneously that morning, while Steven was driving to school he too received a warning from God that this baby would be a "noosling".

Neither of us was surprised at the arrival of our little "noosling". That labor became in a quiet park. I headed home, bathed the children and put them to bed. I called the midwife to give her notice. Then, I called my mother, who was five hours away.

Authentic Health

When the midwife arrived, I was not in hard labor was not breathing heavy, and we sat in this state for quite a while by midnight, she suggested that I was not actually in labor. I knew I was insisted that I would have the baby before my mother arrives in Virginia. The midwife suggested that we all go to bed if labor picked up and we would have a baby is not she would slip out quietly and come back at the appropriate time.

So, at 12:30 midnight. I went to bed, and by 1:30 am within hard heavy labor. I labored briefly in the tub and then got out. I stood next to my bed side pushing Liberty's head out as head emerged the midwife said very calmly, "Try not to push the cord is wrapped." Neither Steve nor I were alarmed as we had been prepared by the Lord earlier that morning. The labor was so fast that another wave of contractions hit immediately and before the midwife could cut the cord from around her neck and she was pushed three of the womb. The proper procedure being to roll the shoulders out of the wrapped cord, which is exactly what we did and she was born.

It was a beautiful birth, very symbolic of the journey of following her birth, through a strangling post partum period, where I felt as if I was dying. I look back now and see that nutritionally I was lacking fats and zinc. But this was part of the journey of discovery.

Solomon's Arrival, " I Got My Brother!"

Solomon was the first of our unassisted or intimate home birth experiences. We had moved the previous year to Missouri. At the time in Missouri midwives were considered "phelons". Literally they could go to prison.

Authentic Health

Ridiculous at that sounds, the medical establishment of that state had such a stronghold on the birthing industry, that unless you knew someone who had had a homebirth it was difficult to find a midwife. There were some licensed midwives but there were 2 in the state and after visiting with one by phone before even becoming pregnant, I knew her frame of reference was much more medically oriented and invasive than mine and that she would not be the person I wanted to attend me. When I found out I was pregnant I was not certain what direction we would go, until a friend suggested delivering unassisted. After talking with Steven about it, we both agreed that this was likely the direction God had for our family. I started reading about unassisted or intimate birth online. During the pregnancy I read several books that really helped solidify that this was the next direction we were to go.

The Power of Pleasurable Childbirth by Laurie Morgan

Unassisted Homebirth: An Act of Love by Lynn Griesemer

After reading these books and the birth stories they recount of many, many women I felt more and more confident with our decision.

I went into labor while at my office around 4:00 pm and drove home. While on the road I called my mom in Virginia, she and my sister-in-law were driving out following birth. I had dinner alone in my room as labor was picking up. Unfortunately, my son had a friend over and my labor just wouldn't move on until the boy left. So around 8:30 he left and labor moved on. This is why I encourage people to make sure there is no unnecessary people present. Any added distraction can delay or slow the labor process. Solomon's labor was wonderful. Very little pain. Lots of deep breathing. And then a baby boy, delivered on hands and knees while holding onto a chair and praying aloud. It was probably the most victorious experience. I felt like I had just ran the winning touchdown. We did it together, it was wonderful. My oldest son, Christian, ten at the time was present also. This was important because he had waited 10 years to have a brother. He was as ecstatic as we were. He kept shouting,"I got my brother; I got my brother!"

Another Brother

My next pregnancy came at what seemed a very bad time in my life. We had just expanded our business to two storefronts, doubling all expenses and increasing headaches with personnel, scheduling and finances, when I discovered that I was pregnant. Oh, if I could turn back time.

I was teaching dance, stretching, exercise and toning classes the entire pregnancy as well as dancing in ministry weekly right up to the 40th week. Then he didn't come, for two more weeks. It was so tiring. I went into labor 3 times each time in the evening, and each morning to wake the next morning without a baby in my arms. The third labor started on a Thursday afternoon, while assembling our playset and I was sure as previous patterns went, we would have a little one by midnight. But instead I endured 12 hours of the most horrendously painful labor. I know for some of you 12 hours seems short, but my labors never went past 6 hours before that birth, but to double the time and triple the intensity was almost more than I might have knowingly endured.

Authentic Health

However, as the night went on I would have 15 minutes of waves of labor, one contraction rolling on top of the previous contraction, then 45 minutes of literally nothing. I would lay quietly wishing to sleep, but knowing that another wave would strike in no time. I kept wondering when it would end.

His head was caught on the pelvic bone, this was keeping him from emerging as well as causing the intense rear labor and unreal pressure to the rectum.

The next morning around 6:30 am I called a midwife I knew, she suggested taking Capsicum as an activator to get labor to regulate. I had not thought of that. When Steven went down to find it, he also found some Blue Cohosh which is also known to stimulate labor.

I had wanted my next and supposedly last baby, to be a girl, Serenity. But as the labor wore on, I looked across my room at a book I had been reading called The Worship Warrior by Chuck Pierce and said aloud, this cannot be my Serenity there is no peace here, this is a warrior. How true that was!

I took 2 capsules of Capsicum and Blue Cohosh; then 15 minutes later I took 2 more and within the half hour labor was in full swing, and within 1 hour I had my baby boy, Joseph Alexander. Shortly after taking and labor regulating, Steven oiled with olive oil the insides and supported the rectum area (only after 15 years of marriage can you communicate these types of needs verbally). Within two pushes he was out and born. Finally!

Following his birth, a prophetic friend said that the birth was symbolic of my mind being caught on something just as his head had been caught on the pelvic bone. She was so right. I had been caught or stopped on the idea that my children were holding me back from whatever success was supposed to be. In truth, my children have been my inspiration. They have inspired me to the success that I am still achieving.

After that birth, due to the extreme trauma to my nervous system, I had no feeling in my feet, particularly my toes for about 4-6 weeks. I also experience bleeding hemorrhoids due to the pressure of the contractions and head. I used Varigone cream and they were completely gone in just 3 days. I had friends who had rough labors with the same effects but their hemorrhoids never healed for months. They didn't know about Varigone.

The Princess is Born

When I became pregnant with Serenity, I was participating in a church wide fast. I was fasting meat and media. I am a very disciplined person so the mental aspects of the fast of meat was conquered within 3 days, and I moved on to juggle the nutritional needs of the family without using meat as a protein source. Unfortunately, I was already pregnant a few days along and unaware that I now needed 3 times the protein to maintain my needs and the placenta that was developing to maintain the new baby.

Everyone in my home enjoyed the fast, they all did well and felt well. Unfortunately, I was not as fortunate. I developed an ulcer and felt horrible. There was also a

Authentic Health

great deal of stress, financial and business during her pregnancy. When she was born it was commented that the placenta showed the stress markers of a smoker's placenta. I of course had not smoked during her pregnancy but the stress we both endured took its toll on us both.

Her birth was the birth of my dreams. I felt great throughout the pregnancy. I had used massage therapy weekly, which greatly reduced stress and physical discomfort.

I decided I would definitely not go over due this time. So 2 days before my due date I took 1 tablespoon of Castor oil in a 4 ounce blueberry smoothie. An hour later I took 1 more tablespoon of Castor oil. Within just a few hours I was having dinner with my family and in labor. It was relaxed. I had wanted my daughters to be present at the previous birth but as it went through the night no one was actually present for the arrival. As the evening went on, the labor gradually intensified.

I had decided on a water birth since soaking in the tub had been so soothing with other births. As the pain intensified, I had decided not to get into the pool until I could do nothing else to alleviate discomfort from the progression of labor. As I entered the pool, I decided to call a few friends that would be praying for a safe delivery. It took just a few minutes and after calling I hung up and with my 4 daughters present, Serenity emerged into the world, with worship music playing in the background. So sweet, Daddy holding my hand and my four daughters greeting their new sister, the littlest princess, Serenity Azana-Jewel. The Lord had given me

Authentic Health

her name on the final day of the 40 day fast; He has said "called forth". –Azana means called forth. The morning before her delivery, her father had prayed over her and spoke to her through my tummy and "called her forth". At that moment I knew that would be her birth day.

I wanted my daughters to know as first hand witnesses that the joy of birth out weights the pains experienced in the process and that they need never fear the most natural process of the birth of a new life.

The Final Arrival –The Flame

Though we, many times thought that we were finished having babies; the Lord had other plans. As I was driving one day, I distinctly heard the Lord say the name, Flame...I knew if there was a name, there was another person on the way to join our family.

After doing a pregnancy test later that day, it was confirmed, that there was indeed another little Anderson. I broke the news to Steven, who had suspected and been asking me for several weeks if I thought I might be pregnant.

So I sent him an e-card announcing that he would be a father again. He read it several times thinking someone was playing a joke on him. He came home strangely excited and not worried or angry. We are not perfect people and unplanned pregnancy has been something thrust upon us and we are not always willing recipients. As we talked about the next Anderson, I told him the name the Lord had given. I told him it didn't have to be the first name. He immediately said if it's a girl, I'd like it

Authentic Health

to be Pneuma, for the Holy Spirit. We never agreed on a boy's name the entire pregnancy and thankfully never had to figure out a permanent male name.

The birth was another water birth. Again, my four older daughters were all in attendance with their father. I had again taken a tablespoon of Castor oil to get things started. I am told most people take a cup to induce labor. A small amount only gently nudges labor if it is time. It is not violent or painful, like the drug inductions in the hospital. It also does nothing if given too early. I was 39 plus weeks along so within a few hours I was in labor and our last treasure was arriving.

Again, the peace in the room and the fellowship of women (my daughters) and the borrowed strength of their father, gave me the confidence and courage to, for the ninth time bring life into the world.

Final thoughts

To summarize, the point of sharing all these experiences: Your peace of mind helps bring a peaceful birth experience. Your belief in yourself and your mate and the love that produced the child you carry will bring you to a place of surrender to the natural process that your body was designed to accomplish. As women we must learn the art of trusting in our ability to bring life and to understand that pain is temporary and purposeful during the birth process. The reward for the work of birth is waiting on the other side of the discomfort. Resisting nature is in itself painful. But partnering with the natural process brings the joy of new life.

Chapter 8: Baby Troubles

This Chapter will help you:

- ✓ Observe and better understand your baby's needs
- ✓ How to's of Planning your Strategy
- ✓ Achieving Your Goals- Begin with the End in Mind

Knowing what you are looking at makes all the difference!

This chapter focuses on the various issues that could arise with a new baby or in the first year. Unfortunately, life has been my greatest teacher, most of the advice shared is from personal experience and is either what we did or should have done.

Day Old Low Blood Sugar

The day following birth is an interesting day. Baby sleeps a great deal and so does mom. However, my ninth child, Pneuma brought about a unique lesson. She was born around 1:30am and of course we both slept through the night. While I had woken around 4am to hear her sweet little sounds, I was so tired and milk had yet to come in, so I didn't put it all together in the wee hours that she might have been hungry.

When I woke up in the morning, she would suckle for a moment then drift off to sleep. This continued throughout the day and by 12:30 pm I texted a midwife to ask if I should be concerned. She said yes, that her blood sugar would be so low that she probably couldn't wake up. She instructed me to give her some milk in a dropper. After several droppers full of warm goat's milk she opened her eyes and came to. Then she nursed and everything was fine from there on.

This story is to alert you to possible problems on the first day. If you have heard this information you may remember in the time when this information is important to your baby.

Dehydration

There are other possible problems you can run into. Another issue while nursing can be dehydration. You can tell if an infant is dehydrated if the fontanel on the top of the head is sunken.

For the most part I don't think that nursed babies need bottled water, however if you have a summer baby you may need to give water or at least give a soaking bath for your infant. Sometimes a cranky baby is nothing more than a baby suffering with dehydrated.

Confusion with day and night

Some infants particularly those born in the middle of the night can have confusion over time of day. When this happens it is best to expose the infant to the sunlight. I always lay my babes in the sunniest room in the house throughout the day. Infants will sleep no matter the lighting, this exposure aids their pineal glands to the

Authentic Health

natural cycles of the day. Noon is the most important time to expose the child to natural sunlight, as this resets the circadian rhythms of the pineal gland and consequently the healing and detoxing rhythms of the child's body.

Another helpful aid for this problem is essential oil of Pine. Put about 10-15 drops of pine oil into a pot of water on the stove and allow pot to simmer. The aroma will help reset the pineal. Pine is also beneficial to the immune system and will help cleanse the air of virus and bacterial toxins that float airborne in a house. This can be kept in the air with an atomizer or diffuser as well to purify air and keep baby's sleep patterns balanced.

Colic—YUCK!

When an infant experiences colic, it is due to the liver not being balanced properly. This is, in my opinion, often due to the cord being cut too soon. In a home delivery, it is uncommon to sever the umbilical cord which connects baby to mother until the cord has completely ceased to pulse. During the time that it is still pulsing mother's body is still doing a necessary function to cleanse baby's blood. Prior to birth the chambers of the heart are actually open and begin closing into a four chambered organ as the cord finishes pulsing. Therefore the baby is not yet completely his own individual organism as someone else is still providing for a biological function of cleansing and oxygenating the blood. When the cord is cut prematurely, colic will manifest. The liver has been hit too soon for that little body to handle. This little person becomes uncomfortable and gassy.

Authentic Health

The simplest solutions include sun exposure, or if baby is born in winter put under a full spectrum or infrared light bulb. Also the herbal combination of Catnip and Fennel liquid can be given ¼ tsp hourly as needed. Also, try closing the ileocecal valve regularly in order to train the valve to close on its own. To do this you will take your hand and find the mid-point between the baby's right hip bone and navel. It is easy to do by placing your thumb on navel and your pinkie on hip bone. The point in the middle where your middle finger gently pushes in or massages will train the valve to close. This is also helpful with reflux.

Reflux

Many babies spit up. Though reports of that nature are common, it should not be a regular occurrence. Out of my nine children only 2 have ever spit up. Felicia spit up twice when she was two days old and my milk came in and she over ate and another child spit up when I had eaten chocolate which didn't agree with him.

This being said, it is not the norm for babies to spit up regularly and certainly not the spit up after every feeding. Most commonly, this is connected again with poor liver or digestive function. If you have a nursed baby, it is possible that the baby is allergic or sensitive to something you are eating. My son had the worst gas ever the first time I ate chocolate after he was born. It was such a horrible night that I didn't eat chocolate the rest of the time I nursed him (almost 11 months after the episode). Foods that will cause the most trouble commonly are wheat, dairy products, corn products and food additives.

Eliminating the food will temporarily aid, but addressing the sensitivity is the best solution. When the body is sensitive or reactive to a food it is actually a sign of a nutrient deficiency. If you can log the foods you are eating and the times the reflux occurs, you can figure out which foods are the causes. Also, you can use muscle response testing. We have a simple to use video available on the subject which will easily enable you to decipher the cause of the reflux. (Contact us to obtain a copy.)

The other cause of reflux can be enzyme deficiency. Proactazyme and Liquid Calcium will fix the problem. When feeding, mix a little of this enzyme in breast milk or formula and give orally along with Liquid Calcium. Another cause of reflux can be a valve not being closed in the stomach. This can be gently massaged, closing the valve and eliminating, or at least lessening the reflux.

Teething

Teething can also trigger many other symptoms that are often addressed with drugs and other unnatural approaches, all because the obvious is over looked.

Some symptoms which are often teething in origin are:
- head ache
- reflux/vomiting
- ear ache
- runny nose

Especially during the first 2 years of childhood, it is just common sense to check for teeth coming in. This is likely the cause of much of parental difficulties with their little ones health.

Liquid Calcium can be given 1 tsp as often as the child would like. I have given my children as much as 3 tsps (1 tbsp) three times daily when cutting teeth. When giving Calcium this frequently we had none of the fussy teething baby symptoms, no fevers etc. And the teeth came in uneventfully in 4 days.

Tantrums

What causes these outbursts that never seem to be at a convenient time? (Usually in front of the neighbors or in the grocery store.)

What is the cause? Simply eliminate the following and you should eliminate the problem. First, address blood sugar levels. Start the morning meal with protein -- eggs for example. This will set the blood sugar levels for the day. A hungry child is a candidate for a tantrum.

As a mother, I try to be constantly aware of the time of the day and meal times approaching. A little prevention makes a big difference in how the family functions. I keep a few apples in my van at all times. That way, if I am delayed in running errands, I can pass out apples to tide us over till we get home.

The next culprit in behavior management is dyes and sugar. Eliminate these two demons as often as possible. I have found that the poorest behaviors seem to follow a church function where koolaid, or some type of dye-filled candy is served. Dyes can cause anything from ADD to a tantrum. These are unnecessary toxins; just eliminate them and avoid all the extra trouble they can cause.

The most likely imbalance that causes frequent tantrums is adrenal fatigue. If you have a child who frequently breaks down into a tantrum over the least thing, this child is probably suffering with weak adrenal gland function. This child needs licorice root. This can be given in liquid if the child is too small to swallow a capsule. I have even given it directly out of the capsule under the tongue. The response is almost instantaneous. I have seen a child go from a fit of screaming and throwing himself on the floor to a completely calm child sitting and quietly preparing to eat his dinner within less than 2 minutes of taking Licorice Root. If the child does have weak adrenals, supplements need to be given for an extended time and on a daily basis.

Won't fall asleep

When a babe has difficulty falling asleep, do a quick check of the obvious and non-obvious. First of course, check the diaper, then give a sip of water. If neither is the case, then the body is likely to be low on protein levels or the baby is hungry. Try giving an egg, or Natures Three and Greenzone mixed with applesauce. If the babe is a newborn or has no teeth, try mom eating extra protein-- eggs or meat. Mom may need extra zinc as well.

Another cause of this problem is related to gas. Something as simple as a trapped burp could be causing the babe enough discomfort to not be able to sleep. Try the following: give a little Catnip & Fennel liquid;

massage the abdomen gently; lift the legs toward the chest gently (this will release a little gas if it is trapped).

Baby Not Satisfied

Sometimes the baby is just not full enough to be satisfied. Often mom is not well hydrated or is not eating enough. Or perhaps the mother's milk is not "creamy" enough to make baby feel full. Breast milk is over 50% fat, this "cream" is like a comfort food for baby. So, if mom has bought into the low fat, no fat lie that she needs to get her figure back instead of nourish her baby, baby may not be getting all the fat that baby's tummy and brain need. You see the baby's brain needs the fat in order to properly develop and function. So, fat is comforting, filling and necessary. Mom should try taking Krill oil, Flax oil, or Super Omegas. These will give mom what she is lacking and fill the "tanks" for baby as well. Also, the herb Marshmallow will enrich the milk, making it more satisfying.

Baby's Can Have Food Allergies Too

Unfortunately, adults as well as babies can develop food sensitivities. It is not uncommon for parents to overindulge in favorite food and cause baby, who is nursing to develop sensitivity to these foods. I recalled while nursing my oldest daughter doing a three-day watermelon fast for cleansing purposes at beginning of watermelon season. While I was enjoying it, she began to develop little water blisters on her hands and torso. After the third day, I suddenly realized that she was allergic to

Authentic Health

the watermelon. After consulting a text book I had studied, I also recognize that the foods that also trigger the similar response were foods that we had been indulging in quite liberally. Foods like rice, cinnamon, and blueberries , which trigger the same allergic response. These were staple foods which we had been greatly enjoying during watermelon season, thus increasing the potential for an allergic reaction. Once I discontinued the watermelon and supplemented my diet with Red Raspberry capsules (the antidote for this allergenic series), the water blisters immediately dried up and disappeared.

The lesson taught me a great deal. That was when I began the practice of food rotation, which I discussed in an earlier chapter. The practice will greatly reduce the incidence of the sensitivity. Food sensitivities in infants can cause anything from the extreme of water blisters or hives to an upset stomach, reflux or excessive discomfort from gas.

When my oldest son was an infant, I recall overindulging in chocolate covered peanuts when he was only a few weeks old. I now know he is severely allergic to peanuts. Now looking back, I am certain the gas that continued all through the night and kept me awake while constantly burping the poor little fellow was a result of the peanuts. At the time I believed it was the caffeine in the chocolate the simulated this but now am certain it was the peanuts. As a teen we discovered he is highly allergic to peanuts, including the oil.

Food rotation will help you identify an offending food fairly quickly. If you chart your food rotation, it will

Authentic Health

simplify great deal. It will enable you to do see what you have been eating as well as to consider what you will be eating. It's easier to make changes when one can clearly identify the offending foods.

Authentic Health

General Nursing

Women often times have difficulties with nursing. The following is a list of possible areas that could be the cause:
- Positioning of baby
- Inverted nipples
- Vitamin C levels
- Lumps – Clogged Ducts
- Breast infections

Check the position of baby on the nipple, if there is any discomfort it is likely that the baby is not in a good centered position on the nipple as you nurse. Also try not allowing baby to nurse endlessly. The breast is generally emptied after 7 minutes on each side. Allowing baby the comfort of suckling, is only adding air to his belly and therefore more gas. Often I would find myself putting my baby to the breast for every little noise when in actuality she needed to burp, sleep, pass gas, or just be changed. Instead I was giving all my reserves to an unwilling dinner guest.

Sounds that Babies make can be interpreted

I actually taught my children to eat to comfort themselves for everything. This is easy to do especially with a bottle baby, when every peep is interpreted as a hunger cry. It is helpful to look at the words or sounds that babies universally know from birth. These sounds were identified by Priscilla Dunstan. Following you will find a Wikipedia link as well as the 5 words and their interpretation. Unfortunately, I was not exposed to this information until my eighth child was born.

Authentic Health

Consequently, the previous children had a different experience. My last two girls were understood much better and therefore not overfed or trained to just eat to pacify themselves.

According to Priscilla Dunstan, there are five universal words (or *sound reflexes*) used by infants worldwide, regardless of language of origin.

Neh-I'm hungry - An infant uses the sound reflex "*Neh*" to communicate its hunger. The sound is produced when the sucking reflex is triggered, and the tongue is pushed up on the roof of the mouth.

Owh-I'm sleepy - An infant uses the sound reflex "*Owh*" to communicate that they are tired. The sound is produced much like an audible yawn.

Heh-I'm experiencing discomfort - An infant uses the sound reflex "*Heh*" to communicate stress, discomfort, or perhaps that it needs a fresh nappy. The sound is produced by a response to a skin reflex, such as feeling sweat or itchiness in the bum.

Eairh-I have lower gas - An infant uses the sound reflex "*Eairh*" to communicate they have flatulence or an upset stomach. The sound is produced when trapped air from a belch that is unable to release and travels to the stomach where the muscles of the intestine tighten to force the air bubble out. Often, this sound will indicate that a bowel movement is in progress, and the infant will bend its knees, bringing the legs toward the torso. This leg movement assists in the ongoing process.

Authentic Health

Eh-I have gas - An infant uses the sound reflex "*Eh*" to communicate that it needs to be burped. The sound is produced when a large bubble of trapped air is caught in the chest, and the reflex is trying to release this out of the mouth

From Wikipedia: http://en.wikipedia.org/wiki/Dunstan_Baby_Language

You can also view this on Dunstan Baby Language DVD.

Authentic Health

Chapter 9: Diet For A Healthy Child

This Chapter will help you:

- ✓ Create A Strategy
- ✓ Understand the How To's Of Creating A Plan
- ✓ Achieving Your Goals- Begin with the End in Mind

Having a Strategy is Half the Battle!

I will not advocate exclusive vegetarian diets. I am not a vegetarian, and quite frankly, I enjoy the abundance and uniqueness of the many foods with which God has blessed the Earth.

I would say in relation to children and their diets, I try to adhere to these principles with my own earthly blessings, that I simply believe that if God didn't make it we shouldn't eat it. My children know when I ask the question, did God make that? Should we eat it? Many times they have come from church functions or other events where I have not been present to help them make wise decisions about their food choices. They will begin to describe the foods offered to them. We usually ask if they think God made that Twinkie or colored drink, etc. They immediately say, "No!" This helps them to begin to learn to make their own wise choices.

Another helpful teaching opportunity is meal preparation time. By teaching them to create a colorful plate presentation, they learn to have diverse foods that consist of many colors and therefore many different nutrients.

When children are trained to eat a flavorless limited variety of foods, their palates become deadened to tasteful, satisfying foods. It is sometimes difficult to make a change in our households when we begin to make healthier choices for our families. However, remember you are making life changing and improving choices for your family in order that they may enjoy better health; more comfortable, happier days; and a longer more productive life. Our human taste buds change every 30 days. This means that every 30 days they will begin to appreciate and even enjoy more of the foods that you are introducing.

I can assure you that these changes are worthwhile. They will give you more time to enjoy the important things in life. A sick child neither has fun nor is fun to be with. You are helping them and yourself to enjoy each other more fully and more often.

A healthy diet is the first step to this end. Simply, eat foods that are fresh, lightly cooked and full of life-giving enzymes. A salad daily during the warmer

Authentic Health

months is a good place to get enzymes and nutrients. Milk is not a good source of calcium. Due to over processing, there is little, if any, usable calcium. If, however, you have a source of fresh goat or cow milk which has not undergone processing, you might enjoy the benefits of the nutrients you wish to obtain. However, green leafy lettuces provide much more usable calcium and a more abundant supply than the milk source.

Chop them finely and incorporate them into Mexican taco salad or in garden salads. Start children on these salad dishes as soon as they have back teeth to chew them with. Even before, when they have their front teeth, the other veggies like carrots, cucumbers, and celery can be introduced. Try serving dried fruits instead of candy. They are much more nutritious. Junk food is extremely costly for fuel that burns quickly and provides little nutrition and therefore does not fill the child's stomach for very long. A nourishing meal lasts for a good while before hunger strikes again.

For recipes and menu plans see my next book, <u>Hey Mom, What's On The Menu</u>? This book can help you plan for healthy nutrition while saving time and money.

The healthy child eats God made food more often than any other type of food. This simply means to eat as many foods in the form God made it. The key

Authentic Health

is limiting the amount of processed foods. These foods are linked with the diabetic epidemic our nation faces today. It is a little known fact that this generation of children faces a life expectancy only into their 50's. Unlike past generations whose life expectancy was in their 70s. Today's generation is likely to die before their parents.

You may wonder how this can be true? There are three specific factors which have brought our society to this point. First, caloric intake has dramatically increased from the intake of our predecessors. Next, the current health model has produced a society of 60 plus percent obese individuals. And the popularity of Corn as a food additive and ingredient has practically made it a food group unto itself.

How can we change these trends? First, let us examine corn intake. To most Americans, corn is recognized as a vegetable. However, it is actually botanically a grain. It grows on a seed head and is therefore a misunderstood plant. It has become one of the most overused foods Americans eat today. It finds itself used as a filler, sweetener, fat and/or binder. It acts like a sweet glue in our systems. In animal feeds corn is always used as a fattener. Consider that, do you want to be fattened, filled, sweetened or bound up? I certainly do not.

So, how do you know what you are feeding your kids? First, you educate yourself on reading labels.

Authentic Health

Understanding the labels and ingredients will greatly assist you in only bringing the best foods into your home and therefore bringing foods which will equip your children's bodies for health.

If we invest the time in choosing the best, we train our children to enjoy the best foods more than the inferior alternatives. We will see future generations' health patterns change and improve. When reading labels, avoid products with: MSG (Mono sodium glutamate); corn and corn derivatives; dyes and color additives; and especially artificial sweeteners. All these ingredients are toxic and known health antagonists.

By avoiding these, you avoid their toxic side effects. You choose the better alternative of authentic health. If you can not buy fresh all the time, then try to buy frozen or canned as alternatives. Frozen is considerably closer to the fresh variety in nutrient content and so would be more beneficial.

Eat From The Pyramid, Look Like A Pyramid

Yes, once again I'm reminding you that the pyramid is not a picture of health. The current model for healthy eating, that our government propagates, includes too many grains and not enough fruits and veggies and far too few fats for healthy glandular or brain and nervous system function. As I mentioned in a previous chapter, it is more important to eat in

Authentic Health

the center. This refers to the idea of eating foods that grow or run. These foods are life-giving as they themselves are alive. The current pyramid model is exactly what has created the diabetic and overweight epidemic we observe today.

Using common sense and lots of variety will make the greatest difference in providing your children a healthy diet. Healthy fats in the form of nuts; seeds; and cold pressed oils, will provide adequate nutrition for the brain, cardiovascular system, glandular organs and skin. Five to seven servings of fruits and vegetables daily will give your child's body plenty of raw nutrients as well as fiber. Avoiding excessive amounts of grains will help the body by not straining the pancreas. Eating adequate protein keeps blood sugar in balance and reduces cravings for junky foods.   Healthy protein includes: fish, turkey, venison and grass fed animals, as well as protein found in nuts,

Chapter 10: Bowel & Digestive Health: Keys to A Peaceful Mind

---

This Chapter will help you:

- ✓ Understand the body's dependence on healthy digestion and elimination
- ✓ Understand how the body's eliminatory system functions best
- ✓ Improve the body's current digestive and bowel health

You are exactly what you digest

The bowels truly are the beginning of all disease processes. Once, after returning from a long trip, our oldest daughter began to experience terrible coughing at night while sleeping. We became increasingly concerned. Finally, on the second night of this coughing, she could not rest. She was not asleep, nor was she awake. She would just cough and whimper as she tried to sleep. We did all the cough remedies (mentioned in chapter cold and flu chapters), but nothing seemed to help. Finally, the answer came. We looked at each other, and I asked my husband if he knew if she had been eliminating in the last two days since returning home. Neither of us could remember helping her wipe up after eliminating. (She was 3 at the time.)

Authentic Health

At that point we went back to the old-fashioned practice of enemas. After three small enemas she passed a number of large clay-like balls the size of large concord grapes. Then during the third enema, she began to pass the vegetables that had been served as her dinner. That was the end of the cough. Immediately, her body relaxed. She stopped coughing and the crisis was over.

What led to this crisis? Several weeks of travel, and therefore, long periods of physical inactivity, which she was also not accustomed to. Also, a poor diet during the final 4 days of our trip that included fast-food because we were museum hopping, and that was all that was available. She was very unaccustomed to such a lifestyle, and therefore, her usual good bowel health was upset. She just couldn't keep up with the digestive and bowel stress. Thus a form of constipation set in, and her body began to give warning signs that dis-ease, or lack of ease, was occurring. After the constipation was alleviated, she immediately had relief of the symptom of coughing.

Remember this story if you have a symptom which does not respond to remedies for that symptom.

Normally, constipation has a simple root in diet, as did the above. First, look at how much pasta, bread, or meat the child is eating. It is probably excessive. These are difficult to digest, and if not accompanied by lots of fresh fruits and vegetables. The child will begin to suffer from constipation.

Constipation is anything less than one elimination per meal. Simply, for every meal eaten there should be a waste product produced within 8-10 hours after the meal

Authentic Health

is eaten. Many times the bowel is clogged as a result of dehydration. Obviously, water is essential. Neither soda, kool aide, juice, tea or coffee will meet the body's need for water. Each human needs half their body's weight in ounces per day. So, if a child weighs 40 pounds, she would need 20 ounces of water each day.

In contrast, the effect of soda, tea, coffee or sugary drinks are actually dehydrating. It takes up to eight times the quantity of water to just break even. For this reason as well as others to be discussed later, sodas should be avoided.

Sometimes children are plagued with dry stools; they will complain of not being able to "push their poops out". This is a dry stool. Chinese Blood Builder is the best formula for this problem. These should be taken as recommended on the bottle for older children or half the dose for younger or smaller children.

If the child is a toddler or infant, you should use Liquid Chlorophyll. Put 1 teaspoon into a few ounces of water. You will begin to see a difference within 24 hours. (The stool will turn green like the Chlorophyll.)

The next cause of constipation is lack of fiber. This form of constipation can be remedied by using a mucilaginous or moisturizing fiber source. Slippery Elm is the simplest to use as it has no flavor and can be stirred into apple sauce or mixed into juice. You can usually expect to see improvement within 24 hours and usually faster.

Authentic Health

Begin by thinking: diet, water and fiber. Then make your remedy selection based on your child's symptoms. The most effective remedy matches the unique situation.

The two extremes of bowel issues are constipation and diarrhea. We have previously discussed the many causes of bowel problems. However, it is important to understand that at the core of bowel difficulties is poor digestion. It is critical to eat foods that are live and fresh so that your body can gain vital nutrition and fiber from the foods being eaten.

Provided you have a strong digestive system, meaning an enzyme rich environment in the stomach, the body will then send the food from the stomach into the small intestine. When it enters the small intestine, it should be the consistency of pureed soup. If soup enters the small intestine, then a healthy elimination will be the product. However, if the bowel receives only a partially digested product, a healthy elimination cannot be the expectation.

So, what makes the foods we eat into soup? First, teach your children to chew thoroughly. Food should leave the mouth almost an unidentifiable mush. Secondly, make sure your children have strong digestive enzymes. Digestive enzymes reduce in strength and quantity naturally after the age of 30. Sometimes due to prolonged poor eating the body will not have proper enzymes to digest certain foods. You can add Proactazyme, which is a plant based enzyme that can even be opened into baby food or baby formula. Many baby formulas have a higher than healthy iron content and can therefore constipate baby. If your baby or child seems to be eliminating poorly, add a capsule of

Authentic Health

Proactazyme to the baby's bottle or into apple sauce. This will help break down the undigested matter.

What is a healthy bowel movement? The following description may be quite shocking to many readers. Most people think an occasional elimination is fine or that a single daily elimination is normal. Sadly, colon cancer is on the rise because of this misinformation. The large intestine or colon is shaped like a large tube of about 2 inches in diameter (in adults). This tube curves roughly from the right hip bone up to bottom of the rib cage across the body to the other side of the rib cage. Then down to the left hip bone and out the rectum.

If you take a tape measure and measure this distance you will find that this is the length of a healthy elimination for your body. In a child, logically, this distance would be shorter and the diameter smaller.

A healthy bowel movement is never ribbon-like or pencil thin. Only in a newborn should the consistency be like liquid. It should also float; not sink. Newly digested matter will float near the surface where as old decaying matter will sink to the bottom. The need for healthy sources of fiber is evident in this observation.

Now, if this is what a healthy elimination looks like, how often should we have one? A simple answer is: how many meals do you eat? If you eat the traditional 3 meals a day, you should have 3 eliminations. For every meal you eat, you can expect a waste product to be formed and eliminated. Remember, if this is not the case, you may need one of the following: enzymes, fiber or water.

Authentic Health

Keys to Healthy Bowels: Things to have on hand

- Proactazyme to break down undigested matter
- Natures Three Fiber (contains the three different types of fiber)or Everybody's Fiber for those with Irritable Bowel
- Purified water (preferable Reverse Osmosis)
- Enema bag or Ear Syringe if you have little children
- Liquid Cleanse formula or LBS II to clear bowels quickly when blocked
- Keep Bentonite Clay to prevent food poisioning and diarrhea

Authentic Health

Homeopathics for Diarrhea

Argentum nitricum: If a person has diarrhea when anticipating a stressful event (such as giving a speech or a public performance, taking a test, or attending a party), this remedy should come to mind. Bloating and flatulence are usually seen, pain may be felt in the region of the groin, and the diarrhea may look green. Diarrhea that occurs immediately after eating or drinking, or after eating too much sugar, will often respond to *Argentum nitricum*.

Arsenicum album: Diarrhea accompanied by anxiety, restlessness, and exhaustion suggest a need for this remedy. Burning pain is felt in the digestive tract and the person may be thirsty for frequent small sips of tea or water. The stools may be watery and have a putrescent odor. Simultaneous diarrhea & vomiting is another strong indication. *For food poisoning.*

Bryonia :This remedy is often helpful for diarrhea during flu (especially when grumpy and wants to lie still and be left alone). It may also be helpful for diarrhea that occurs when a person gets overheated; then drinks a lot of cold water. Symptoms often are worse in the morning. The person's mouth may be very dry.

Chamomilla: Hot, green, watery diarrhea with abdominal pain and gas suggests a need for this remedy. The person's face will be red and flushed (sometimes only on one side) and problems may be worse from warmth. Children who need this remedy will often seem extremely angry, & scream or hit. Adults are irritable & hypersensitive.

Colocynthis: Cutting and cramping pains in the abdomen precede the diarrhea when this remedy is indicated. The person feels relief from doubling over, or from putting hard pressure on the abdomen. This remedy is often helpful when diarrhea follows anger (especially if the feelings were not expressed).

Gelsemium: This remedy is often indicated if trembling & weakness accompany diarrhea, especially when nervousness, fear, or emotional upset is the cause. *Gelsemium* is also useful during flu with diarrhea, droopy lethargy, fever, chills, and headache.

Ipecacuanha: If a person has diarrhea accompanied by extreme or constant nausea, this remedy may bring relief. Cutting, clutching pains are worse around the navel, and the diarrhea looks frothy or green.

Phosphorus: This remedy can be soothing if a person has a weak or empty feeling in the abdomen, followed by diarrhea that runs out "like an open faucet." People who need this remedy are often thirsty, and may be fearful when ill.

Podophyllum: Profuse, gushing, watery diarrhea that is usually not accompanied by pain suggests the use of this remedy. The abdomen rumbles and gurgles before the diarrhea passes, and urging may soon be felt again. Bouts of diarrhea are often worse in the morning, and also in hot weather.

Pulsatilla: If diarrhea occurs after eating rich and fatty foods, this remedy can be helpful. Queasiness and abdominal pain are likely to occur and the diarrhea has a changeable appearance. The person usually is not thirsty, feels worse from being warm or in a stuffy room; and is better in open air. A need for attention, sympathy, and comforting is a strong indication for *Pulsatilla* (a very useful remedy for children).

Sulphur: Urgent, hot diarrhea that occurs in the early morning, making the person rush to the bathroom, suggests a need for this remedy. Burning is often felt in the digestive tract, and the anus can be itchy, red, and irritated. The person may also have hemorrhoids that burn and itch.

Homeopathics for Constipation

Bryonia: For constipation with a feeling of dryness in the rectum and large dry stools that are hard to push out, with sticking or tearing pains. The person feels grouchy or out of sorts, and may be tense from business-related worries.

Calcarea carbonica: People who need this remedy often feel more stable when constipated, and experience discomfort and fatigue when the bowels have moved. Large stools are hard at first, then sticky, then liquid. The person may feel chilly and sluggish, have clammy hands and feet, crave sweets, and feel weak and anxious when ill or overworked.

Causticum: Helpful when stool is difficult to pass, with lots of painful straining. The person's face may turn red from effort, and more success may come from standing up. When it finally emerges, the stool will be narrow and full of mucus.

Graphites: This remedy is indicated when large stools look like "sheep dung" or little balls stuck together with mucus. Aching often is felt in the anus after the bowels have moved. People who need this remedy are slow to become alert in the morning, usually stout, and have a tendency toward eczema.

Lycopodium: A person who needs this remedy has frequent indigestion with gas & bloating, & many problems involving the bowels. Rubbing the abdomen or drinking something warm may help to relieve the symptoms. A craving for sweets and an energy slump in late afternoon & early evening are strong indications for *Lycopodium*.

Nux vomica: "Wants to but can't" is a phrase that brings *Nux vomica* to mind. This remedy is often helpful to people who are impatient, tense, and ambitious—who work too hard and exercise too little; indulge in stimulants or alcohol; and are partial to sweets and spicy food. Headaches, chilliness, and constricting pains in the bowels or rectal area often accompany constipation when *Nux vomica* is needed.

Sepia: A heavy sensation in the rectum, remaining after a bowel movement, may indicate a need for this remedy. Stools can be hard and difficult to pass, although they may be small. The person often has cold hands and feet, and is weary and very irritable. Exercise may bring improvement, both to constipation and to mood and energy level. (*Sepia* is often useful to women who develop constipation just before or just after a menstrual period.)

Authentic Health

Silicea (also called Silica): The person strains for long periods without success. A "bashful" stool begins to come out, but eventually retreats. People who need this remedy are nervous and mentally acute, but also chilly, physically frail, and easily fatigued.

Sulphur: Dry, hard stools with reddish inflammation of the anus and offensive flatulence suggest a need for this remedy. Constipation may also alternate with diarrhea. People who need this remedy are often "characters" with interesting mental notions, slouching posture, and very little interest in tidiness.

Chapter 11: Food Allergies & Their Effect on Daily Health

This Chapter will help you:

✓ how digestive health is connected to allergies
✓ how digestive health is connected to behavior
✓ recovering from food sensitivities

Understanding how digestion is connected to food allergies

Many children suffer with endless allergies to this or that. Hay fever, rag weed, etc. seem to plague everyone these days. What are allergies and how are they affecting us? And, lastly how can we fight and win this battle.

First, allergies are nothing more than intolerance to a chemical substance. This intolerance manifests as sneezing, mucous production, respiratory difficulties or a skin reaction, like itching or hives.

So why do some people have such strong intolerance? According to Dr. Lepore in <u>Ultimate Healing Systems</u>, allergens all have antidotes: herbs, vitamins, minerals, or amino acids, as the allergy reaction itself is simply a sign of nutritional deficiency in the individual.

The most common allergens in our society are those to corn, wheat, and dairy. Though there are others like potatoes or other food sources, the above three are the most commonly found allergen reactors. Along with the wheat series sensitivity a person will find sensitivities to dust mites, animal dander, and dust and pollens if sensitive to wheat.

Sadly, the use of decongestants and antihistamines instead of supporting the liver and respiratory system creates greater reactivity in the future. And is the route most parents will use due to a lack of understanding of the real causes of these respiratory allergies.

Simple respiratory support can be found by using ALJ in liquid or capsules. This helps with congestion and lung support. Milk Thistle and Dandelion aid in supporting the liver. Skin reactions can be aided by taking Oregon Grape. Many children and adults with allergies have clogged and congested colons as well. Liquid Cleanse can help clear and clean the colon and help speed the process of alleviating the allergies. When you know what your child reacts to you can then nourish and support them nutritionally in order to alleviate the allergy altogether.

For example, when my oldest daughter was a few months old, watermelon season came along. With the watermelons, came the season for strawberries, blueberries, and other wonders of God's creation. I was eating them and fully enjoying them. But my new baby was nursing exclusively. She was at the mercy of my dietary choices. However, I was enjoying them a little too heartily. I even did a two-day watermelon fast. By the third day, my little baby had little water blisters coming up all over her body. They would burst; I would sprinkle Goldenseal on them, and they would go away. Then, another would show up soon after. I had no idea what might be causing it. Then, a friend suggested that it might be a food allergy. She said her son had done something similar when she ate peaches while nursing.

With this information, I consulted a chart found in Dr. Lepore's book and found that almost all the foods I had been indulging in were in the same food reactivity series. The antidote was a simple herb, Red Raspberry.

Sometimes you must get Personal

Recently, my oldest daughter who has been highly allergenic to corn since she was eight, experienced an allergic response beyond any she had experienced previously. Her eyes swelled, her breathing became very difficult, and sleeping was almost impossible. Unfortunately, when all this happened she was away from home.

In the middle of the night, I received a text stating that she had been up all night unable to sleep, eyes itching, and breathing raspy at best. I immediately suggested she take Sinus Support and Histablock (two of each). This allowed her to get back to sleep. However, the swelling of her eyes did not recede until the next day. Then I sent her a personalized homeopathic remedy, to take. This remedy was personalized to her unique situation. Within 30 minutes of taking it the eyes began to go back to normal and within two hours, her eyes were completely back to their normal state. Now instead of an Epi-Pen , as most people carry, she carries her personal homeopathic. She takes one pellet of that 100C potency along with the specific remedies, which her body needed to overcome the allergic response. And now she is symptom free. In her case she was allergic to corn, wheat and oats, indicating and Iodine, Magnesium and Iron deficiency. With very specific supplementation, these reactions have completely stopped. However, it takes only a few days of indulging in these foods and missing her supplements before she can bring about the same negative symptoms.

Getting to the root of the actual problem and relieving the symptoms from their origins makes all the difference. When an allergic response strikes speed and accuracy in finding the remedy can be critical to a quick healing response.

Chapter 12: The Respiratory System

This chapter will help you understanding signs & significance of the following:

- ✓ Upper Respiratory Seasonal Allergies vs Infection
- ✓ Three Types of Asthma
- ✓ Ear Ache, Runny Nose, Sore Throat
- ✓ Bronchial Infections & Pneumonia

The Digestive Connection

Most respiratory problems begin with a weakened digestive system. If the digestive system is repaired, most allergens are no longer harmful. For example, a fat allergy caused by milk fats could manifest as swollen lymph glands and ear aches or itchy ears. This is simply due to a sulfur deficiency and fat allergy. Simply giving a regular dose of MSM or garlic oil gel cap for children would make all the difference to correcting and eventually eliminating the reactivity all together.

Authentic Health

Dealing with Season Allergies vs Respiratory Infections

The respiratory system can be broken down in to two distinct parts, upper and lower. Upper involves the nose, ears and throat. The lower involves the lungs and bronchial tissue.

The Nasal cavity can be involved in sinus infections or congestion due to seasonal allergies. Seasonal allergies can easily be dealt with by adding strong warming herbs to the digestive system. Horseradish, ginger, garlic and onions are all examples of such things. The formula ALJ is an allergy formula which easily decongests, or opens up the respiratory channels. This formula contains warming herbs which act like a natural Sudafed. As a side benefit, it also helps clear obstructions from nasal passages and lung passages.

If drainage comes predominantly during the night and drains down the back of the throat, or you are experiencing sinus headaches, you should use Sinus Support Formula. This formula stops the drainage while you sleep and clears infection. It also opens sinus passages so that breathing can better take place.

If you are experiencing coughs, colds, and congestion, you should use the formula CC-A. This is great for both adults and children. It boosts vitamin C levels which aids in the histamine response. This formula also breaks down the destructive elements which are causing the congestion and coughing while also clearing mucous.

Authentic Health

Homeopathy for seasonal allergy symptoms

Allium Cepa: Certain pollen allergies cause watery eyes and burning nasal discharge. Sneezing happens but may not be constant. There may be pain in the forehead. People with these type of conditions feel better when they are inside the house in a cool room. They feel worse in warm rooms or in cold weather. Hot foods and drinks make them feel bad as well.

Arsenicum Iodatum: Another type of allergy makes people sneeze constantly followed by an irritation cough. Nostrils are sore and red from the constant sneezing. The throat may also burn. Asthma may accompany the allergy. People with this type of allergy feel worse from sneezing and warm areas.

Euphrasia: Another instance of allergy affects people primarily in the eyes. Eyes are swollen and sensitive to bright light. Eyes are watery. There is little discharge from nose. The mucus drips to the back of the throat. People generally feel better by resting and sleeping. Warm weather and hot areas make this allergy feel worse. Being indoors and out in the evening makes the allergy feel worse.

Sabadilla: this type of allergy causes a sore throat. Swallowing is painful. Eyes are red, swollen, & watery. The throat is very dry. Headaches feel like the head is shrinking. You feel better from eating & drink hot foods and drinks; and worse from cold weather & cold drinks.

Help for 3 Types of Asthma

If the body has difficulty breathing to the point of asthma you would want to open bronchials while clearing the obstruction. The specific herb for this job is Lobelia. It is best used in liquid form. This herb will open the bronchials while also clearing the obstructive matter. When using this herb you may actually expel the mucous through the mouth or bowel.

In the case of asthma, there can be 3 different causes: exercise-induced; stress-induced; chemical-induced or environmentally triggered asthma. All are benefited by Lobelia essence.

However, understanding the cause is as important as locating the cure. Exercise induced asthma actually stems from weakened adrenals. By supporting the adrenals and lungs, you will begin to better oxygenate. In order to do this, the body will need Lobelia essence, Bronchial Formula to strengthen bronchial dilation, and NutriCalm or B-Complex to strengthen the adrenal glands, for younger children use Licorice Root extract.

The second cause of asthma can be stress. When a person's asthmatic attack occurs following bad or sad news the asthma is stress-induced. Again, Lobelia is advised. It acts not only as a de-abstruent but also acts as a nervine or calming element. Skeletal Strength and NutriCalm are both especially helpful for this type of condition as they support the nervous system when under stress and in repairing from past stressors.

The last form of asthma is chemical or environmentally induced. This would occur when you go through the candle or detergent aisle at the grocery store. If breathing difficulty occurs when exposed to these type of substances, then a liver detox to correct the long term issue that has caused the situation. Using Histablock or Milk Thistle Combination would be advisable. Also, use the Lobelia essence to open and clear obstructions that the body has been unable to throw off. Also, use EnviroDetox to clear the body of environmental toxins, which have lodged in any of the eliminatory channels.

Homeopathy for Asthma Attacks

Aconitum Napellus: is one of the top **homeopathic asthma remedies** for attacks which are sudden and moderate to severe. This remedy is also helpful for asthma caused by cold air, such as being outside during winter.
Arsenicum Album: is one of the natural remedies for asthma that can be used in many different situations. It can help with asthma that is acute or chronic, especially with cases where breathing difficulty worsens when lying down and improves when sitting up.
Carbo Vegetabilis: is used as a homeopathic treatment in cases where the individual has a lot of gas and digestive problems, as well as asthma. Sitting up may relieve some of the breathing ability, and burping may also help.
Chamomilla: is one of the homeopathic asthma remedies used when there is a cough that is dry and very irritating. These cases usually involve asthma triggered by excitement or anger, or by moving air.

Ipecacuanha: this helps with excess mucous as well as gagging Ipecacuanha is often used. Vomiting and extreme coughing spasms may also be present during the asthma attack.

Kali Carbonicum: this remedy is used for asthma sufferers who seem to be cold or chilly all the time, such as in cardiac asthma cases where the blood flow is not sufficient. Sitting up in a forward position may also help relieve some pressure from the lungs, and make breathing easier.

Natrum Sulphuricum: This remedy is used for asthma attacks that are triggered by bad weather or cold temperatures.

Nux Vomica: can be a natural alternative to asthma medications over the counter. This remedy is used when asthma results in a tight chest combined with digestive upset. These cases may have the most severe asthma in the mornings.

Pulsatilla: If your asthma gets worse as the day goes by then Pulsatilla may offer relief. These attacks will usually include mucous which is yellow and thick, and choking or gagging during coughing is common.

Spongia Tosta: is one of the homeopathic asthma remedies use when there is little mucous produced and the cough is dry, and sounds similar to barking.

Ears, Nose and Throat

Earaches and sore throats are probably the two most common complaints of children and adults. Again, it is common that the body is actually allergic to something that has been eaten. An example of this would be ice cream. The child eats a cone of ice cream and immediately begins coughing and later develops a sore throat and cough. This is a sign of a food allergy, probably to fats or milk in the ice cream.

Sadly, most parents continue to feed their children such delights on a regular basis. So, it is not a "sometimes food", but rather a daily food. This is where the difficulty comes in. As the body continually intakes these difficult to digest, mucous-producing foods, it builds up mucous in order to protect itself from the toxicity of the food. Consequently, the body has more drips and draining. Adding more dietary sulfur will alleviate this sensitivity.

What if the problem goes on for a prolonged time? Earache and sore throat are surely to ensue. To relieve earaches use CBG Extract directly in to the ears or you can take orally as well. Putting this into the ears will clear infection as well as act a nervine to ease pain and discomfort.

Silver Shield liquid can also be used in ears, gargled and swallowed for sore throat. If a season of extreme unexplainable respiratory congestion occurs, I drink 1 ounce of Silver Shield hourly. I usually feel drowsy and sleep for several hours and feel amazingly recovered following this immune boost.

Authentic Health

If you tend toward these types of respiratory ailments you should also consider taking a daily dose of Nature's Immune Stimulator to keep immune system strong and on guard to potential environmental attacks.

Bronchial Infection and Pneumonia

If you struggle with reoccurring bronchial infection or pneumonia, you likely need to strengthen immune function, while detoxifying and rebuilding lung and bronchial tissue. A maintenance protocol to prevent this type of recurring situation would be the following:

Black Walnut, Bronchial Formula, Marshmallow, and Mullien along with Nature's Immune Stimulator: Together they will improve infection fighting capabilities, open and clear bronchials of debris, moisturize lung tissues and clear mucous and airborne antagonists to your health.

Homeopathics for Bronchitis

Antimonium tartaricum: This remedy is indicated when the person has a feeling of wet mucus in the chest, and breathing makes a bubbly, rattling sound. The cough takes effort and is often not quite strong enough to bring the mucus up, although burping and spitting may be of help. The person may feel drowsy or dizzy, and feel better when lying on the right side or sitting up.
Bryonia: This remedy is often indicated when a cough is dry and very painful. The person feels worse from any movement, and may even need to hold his or her sides or press against the chest to keep it still. The cough can make the stomach hurt, and digestion may be upset. A

very dry mouth is common, and the person may be thirsty. A person who wants to be left alone when ill, and not talked to or disturbed, is likely to need *Bryonia*.

Calcarea carbonica: This remedy is often indicated for bronchitis after a cold. The cough can be troublesome and tickling, worse from lying down or stooping forward, worse from getting cold, and worse at night. Children may have fever, sweaty heads while sleeping, and be very tired. Adults may feel more chilly and have clammy hands and feet, breathing problems when walking up slopes or climbing stairs, and generally poor stamina.

Causticum: Bronchitis with a deep, hard, racking cough can indicate a need for this remedy. The person fees that mucus is stuck in the throat and upper chest, and may cough continually to try to loosen it. A feeling of rawness and soreness can develop, or a sensation as if a rock is stuck inside. Chills can occur along with fever. Exposure to cool air aggravates the cough, but drinking something cold can help. Feel worse when days are cold and clear, and better in wet weather.

Dulcamara: When a person easily gets ill after being wet and chilled (or when the weather changes from warm and dry to wet and cool) this remedy may be indicated. The cough can be tickly, hoarse, and loose, and worse from physical exertion. Tendencies toward allergies (cats, pollen, etc.) may increase the person's susceptibility to bronchitis.

Hepar sulphuris calcareum: The cough that fits this remedy is usually hoarse and rattling, with yellow mucus coming up. The person can be extremely sensitive to cold—even a minor draft or sticking an arm out from under the covers may set off jags of coughing. Cold food or drink can make things worse. A person who needs this remedy feels vulnerable both physically and emotionally, and may act extremely irritable and out of sorts.

Kali bichromicum: A metallic, brassy, hacking cough that starts with a troublesome tickling in the upper air-tubes and brings up strings of sticky yellow mucus can indicate this remedy. A sensation of coldness may be felt inside the chest, and coughing can lead to pain behind the breastbone or extending to the shoulders. Breathing may make a rattling sound when the person sleeps. Problems are typically worse in the early morning, after eating and drinking, and from exposure to open air. The person feels best just lying in bed and keeping warm.

Pulsatilla: Bronchitis with a feeling of weight in the chest, and a cough with choking and gagging that brings up thick yellow mucus, may respond to this remedy. The cough tends to be dry and tight at night, and loose in the morning. The fever may be worse in the evening and at night. Feeling too warm or being in a stuffy room tends to make the person worse, and open air brings improvement. Thirst is usually low. A person who needs this remedy often is moody and emotional and wants attention and sympathy. (This remedy is often helpful to children who are tearful when not feeling well and want to be held and comforted.)

Authentic Health

Silicea (also called Silica): bronchitis for weeks at a stretch, or even all winter long. The cough takes effort and may bring up yellow or greenish mucus, or little granules that have an offensive smell. Stitching pains may be felt in the back when the person is coughing. Chills are felt more than heat during fever, and the person is likely to sweat at night. A person who needs this remedy is usually sensitive and nervous, with low stamina, swollen lymph nodes, and poor resistance to infection.

Sulphur: Is indicated when a person has had many bouts of bronchitis (sometimes the resistance has been weakened by taking antibiotics too often for minor complaints). The cough feels irritating, burning, and painful; yellow or greenish mucus may be produced. Problems can be worse if the person gets too warm in bed, and breathing problems at night may wake the person up. Redness of the eyes and mucous membranes, and foul-smelling breath and perspiration are often seen.

Clearing Triggers Can be Key

Identifying Trigger factors can help bring about healing faster

- Environmental concerns
- Dietary concerns
- Emotional performance
- Insufficient rest
- Insufficient water
- Bacterial or viral concerns

Your environment can greatly affect your respiratory health. For example, new carpet can introduce allergic reactions to plastics. An ozonator or air purification system may be your only solution in a home filled with new carpet. Heavy reactivity to plastic or unnatural goods should be addressed with the EnviroDetox and Bronchial formula, along with Lobelia essence if necessary. When the person is extremely allergic to plastics, the liver is highly toxic and should be addressed with Milk Thistle Combination.

The diet can obviously be a large part of the stress which triggers respiratory concerns. As mentioned in the previous chapter, these can be addressed by different supplements to correct certain reactionary substances. Refer to the previous chapter for more information.

Believe it or not, ongoing emotional upset can be a trigger for respiratory difficulties. Everyone knows that when they are grieving the lungs and sinuses weep. When there is a chronic long term respiratory issue, it is good to consider what has been going on in life that could be upsetting you. Begin to pray and seek God's guidance as to how to resolve the issue that is stealing your health. Ask God to bring back joy and gladness in exchange for your sorrow and sadness.

Basic Quick Respiratory Tips to Stop Breathing Problems in their tracts

Always have on hand the following Food:

- Almonds as they help improve breathing
- Honey as it is a natural soothing element for sore throats and congestion
- Onions as they clear lymph, congestion and mucous

Authentic Health

- Lemons as they promote immune function and improve painful throats

Stop Coughing with these remedies

Mix the following together and take liberally as needed to soothe coughing:

- 10 drops Tei Fu oil
- 1 Tsp honey
- ¼ tsp of Lobelia Essence

Rub Tei Fu oil or Massage lotion liberally on the bottoms of feet and cover with socks. This will greatly reduce coughing and allow you to rest and heal.

Soak the feet in a hot foot bath with minced onions.

Heat onions in the oven till juicy then place on a thin cloth on top of the neck, chest and back to break down congestion and mucous.

Place a heating sack or hot water bottle on top of onion poultice in order to keep warm longer.

Onions can also be used topically on the ear for an ear infection as well.

Chapter 13: The Nervous Connections: ADD, Slow Learning, Ticks, Stuttering, Eye Sight

Understanding the Nervous System and Triggers to Downed Wires:

- ✓ Food Allergen Connections
- ✓ Vaccine Connections
- ✓ Feeding and Maintaining for maximum healing and efficiency

ADD & ADHD...The Tragedy of our Youth

ADD and ADHD are some of the most over diagnosed problems plaguing our children today. The plague is not the condition but rather the diagnosis. Many people have a general practitioner, or even a school teacher randomly identify your child with this label. Sadly, neither of these people have enough background to label these children as ADD or ADHD. This is a psychiatric diagnosis and only a licensed psychiatrist can actually diagnose this problem. And this diagnosis is only after lengthy diagnostic evaluations. Unfortunately, the general practitioner does have the right to write a prescription for psychiatric drugs such as Ritalin and other mind-altering drugs.

Authentic Health

As parents are unaware that these drugs are class III narcotics equal are equal to the affect in many ways in the brain as the illegal drug heroin. Most branches of the military do not accept young people who have been on these drugs because they are aware of the long-term psychiatric affects. These drugs cause infertility in male children if taken before older teen years. Children who have been on these and/or antidepressants are known to have significantly higher rates of suicide before the age of 18.

Sadly, many parents who lack time, or basic training in parenting skills, choose to subject their children to dangerous drugs in order to control behavior they neither understand, nor attempt to work through. It is my opinion that most children with ADD, like symptoms, simply need more attention, plus one-on-one time with parents and other caring adults. Unfortunately, in modern society it is much simpler to give a pill than give our time to our children. These young people, I believe, if left un-medicated and given proper training and praise, would be the geniuses of tomorrow. Instead, a society chooses to medicate this generation of geniuses and hide the brilliance within a high energy person. Trapped in the presence of medication, they are unable to release all of the beauty and creativity that God placed within them.

Authentic Health

Eliminating some triggers to Behavioral Outbursts

There are many substances which can trigger or unleash these poor behaviors. As discussed in the previous chapter on Food Allergens, foods can be a trigger substance. These foods need not be junk food or sugary substances. They can be simply a food the child consumes that sets off a chain of events that leads to nervous system overload. This triggers the adrenals to misfire and begin a chain of outburst like behaviors.

Corn Syrup and corn bi-products, in my opinion, is the most frequent culprit in our American diets today. So many, in fact most, food products contain some type of corn bi-product. Our animal feeds are laden with corn and therefore , our diets are saturated with corn. From observation, I would say that corn is a primary trigger substance for many young people.

Dyes and Sugar

The next culprit in behavior management is dyes and sugar. Eliminate these two demons as often as possible. I have found that the poorest behaviors seem to follow a church function where koolaid, or some type of dye filled candy. Dyes can cause anything from ADD to a tantrum. These are unnecessary toxins, just eliminate them and avoid all the extra trouble they can cause.

I would suggest that if you have some of these problems, you begin with diet changes and perhaps lifestyle changes. The first change is to eliminate toxic and stressful chemicals from the diet. For example, begin by removing all food colorings. Red, Yellow, and Blue Dyes are some of the worst and most quickly reacting chemicals. My daughter could have a snack at church with food coloring and bounce off the wall for a couple of hours. Even bubble gum with coloring on the outside would send her off. These dyes can also cause bedwetting. Beware of the potential hazards of allowing your children to enjoy these highly reactive toxins.

With these changes, you may begin seeing a change in behavior. You cannot imagine how many foods that you don't even realize have dyes, most cereals, many cheeses, cookies, most cake mixes, some breads, yogurt, ice cream, many juice drinks, koolaide, Gatorade, and sodas. Eliminating these foods and drinks will make a dramatic difference in your child. A Homeopathic Detox Protocol may be necessary and helpful. You can order this by contacting me by email (listed at the end of the book).

MSG, or MonoSodiumGlutamate

The next substance to eliminate is MSG, also known as MonoSodiumGlutamate. This can cause everything from panic attacks to seizures and tantrums. In adults, this chemical can trigger heart attacks, swelling, headaches and panic attacks as well. Read your labels and eliminate this problem quickly. As a young girl, I used to have panic attacks after eating Campbell's soup. The Campbell's soups contain MSG except for the low-sodium recipe at this time.

Supplements and Foods to Feed the Brain and Nervous System

These measures should succeed in making a dramatic improvement in your child's ability to focus, but there is also an effective herbal protocol which follows:

Nature's Chi is a supplement which acts like a natural Ritalin in the body without altering personality, educational ability, or creativity. It helps the child to have a natural calm and direction. This used along with Focus Attention will enable the child to stay on task. B-Complex can also be useful with those individuals who struggle with attention disorders. Flax Seed Oil or Super Omegas are also important because the body and brain need fats to help the brain give these supplements prior to leaving for school with breakfast.

Another important aspect of these problems is of course nutrition. Beginning the day with a protein breakfast like eggs, and even in some cases even using steak with the eggs, helps balance blood sugar and eliminates hypoglycemic blood sugar fluctuations. These fluctuations can cause the child to act out or become distracted from studies.

Determining glandular imbalances

It it's not uncommon that a low thyroid function or weak adrenal gland can be triggered for behavior and horrible outbursts. Below are listed the symptoms and solutions for these chronic causes of poor behavior.

Authentic Health

Weak adrenals.

When the adrenals are low is not common to see tantrums as discussed before. Other symptoms are as follows:

- Inability to face the sun; squinting the eyes.
- Constant craving for sugar.
- Energy lows between 10 &11 am &1 & 2pm.
- Depression and anxiety.

Low thyroid function

- Fatigue and Sluggishness or Depression
- Increased sensitivity to cold
- Constipation
- Pale, dry skin or A puffy face
- Hoarse voice
- An elevated blood cholesterol level
- Unexplained weight gain or loss
- Muscle aches, tenderness and stiffness
- Pain, stiffness or swelling in your joints
- Muscle weakness
- Heavier than normal menstrual periods
- Brittle fingernails and hair

If you're seeing any of the above symptoms it is important to address them now rather than wait until the body completely breaks down. Some simple solutions are easily at hand. As we discussed earlier Licorice Root is very beneficial to the adrenals. Herbs such as Spirulina, Black Walnut, and Thyroid Activator are extremely beneficial formulas for a poorly functioning thyroid.

Slower Learners, Low IQ and Stuttering

Many times low intelligence is actually an under-nourished thyroid and brain. This can happen during the pre-birth or gestational development, but it can also be a result of poor diet after birth.

In recent studies it has conclusively been shown that breast-fed babies grow into higher IQ adults. The study also showed that the length of nursing needed to be at least 9 months. This is also a boost to the immune health of your child forever.

Also, be aware that your body's strengths and weaknesses will also be in your milk's chemical make-up. That means that if you are deficient in some nutrient, for example iodine, you will also pass this lack on to your infant. I suggest that while nursing you supplement your own diet with Herbal Trace Minerals. I also suggest using Mineral Chi Tonic. Both of these will give you vital trace minerals and immune support for you and your child. You will also be supporting your pituitary, thyroid and liver. These are the three most taxed organs and glands when you are pregnant. This helps with your recovery and helps baby to stay strong as well. Again, the brain and thyroid are usually the weak links when there is a case of low intelligence. You can also use Spirulina to aid in RNA & DNA problems like autism, retardation, etc.

Authentic Health

Stuttering

Many children have problems with stuttering and their parents really don't know why or what to do for it. However, there is much to do for it. Stuttering is simply a delay in the synapse of the brain. The child has information he wants to share, but the synapse is delayed and not transmitted clearly or timely.

What can a mother do? First, build the thyroid. Why the thyroid? The thyroid controls metabolic energy or speed at which nutrients are released to the vital organs. In this case, the brain is the vital organ. The nutrients needed for the brain to not only survive but thrive, are found in such herbs as Black Walnut extract. This is a liquid and can be taken straight or mixed in juice. I suggest taking it straight simply for the fact that you know your child has taken all that you intended him to have.

I have seen a child go from stuttering in every sentence he spoke to no stuttering at all in two weeks time. I have also seen children who were very late talkers begin talking in about two days from this program as well. The other supplements that I would recommend to build and strengthen brain function which will enable the child to perform more efficiently in speech areas are GABA, and Flax Seed Oil or Super Omegas.

You will be simply amazed at the progress your child will make in a short period of time with just the consistency that you can provide. Take all of these supplements twice daily to improve brain function, speed of thinking, eliminate stuttering and improve learning.

Authentic Health

Poor Vision, Crossed or Lazy Eyes

Additionally, it should also be noted that poor vision is also linked to poor thyroid function. If your child has poor vision at an early age, it is important to supplement the thyroid and nervous system. I have seen children at age 5 with bottle thick glasses. Within a three month time of supplementation, this same child has improved his vision to the point that his eye doctor could not explain the improvement. He had also improved his scores in his classroom dramatically. Where the eye doctor had previously been suggesting eye surgery for young child he was now lowering the prescription of his glasses.

Lazy or Crossed eyes are also connected with a struggling thyroid. Remember that the brain is fed leftovers from the thyroid, so the two are linked. If the brain is not fed well, specifically iodine, stuttering, and vision issues can manifest. Incorporate Black Walnut and Focus Attention by opening capsule into apple sauce, yogurt or oatmeal. Along with Flax Seed oil to strengthen the nerves , you should see noticeable improvement within a month. Continued supplementation can correct the situation.

Chapter 14:
The Vaccine Connection

Vaccine Damage, Yes it is possible and probable.

- ✓ Just think logically
- ✓ Understanding your legal parental rights

Do your research...YOURSELF

Many books have been written on this topic. These books contain far more informative details than I will choose to give on this subject. I choose only to address this topic from a logical and spiritual perspective.

I would pose a question. Would you serve your child a glass of formaldehyde, mercury, or puss from the kidney of a dead monkey? I feel certain that your answer is an emphatic, "NO!" If you wouldn't serve it in a glass or on a platter, why would you forcibly bypass the body's natural defenses of the skin or digestive system and inject it into your little precious baby's body?

Sounds quite crazy, but people do it every day. Why? It's quite simple really, the "Great Doctor" (who they have given the power of God; that of life and death) has told them to do this.

I suggest that as a society, we might really take the opportunity to inform ourselves better about the side effects we are experiencing from these poisons. If you would not serve it for dinner, should you break through the body's natural defense, "the skin" and force a known toxic poison into the body's immune system? The logic that this therefore causes the body to build up immunity that it formerly lacked to various viruses is as logical as saying that through daily beatings your child will grow to someday be able to withstand the beatings that he/she may someday endure at the hands of a psychopath.

What kind of preparation and at what cost is this type of "prevention?" These substances have known side effects and are known poisons. However, together they are considered by our medical community to contain some mysterious preventive healing ability. The mere thought does sound ludicrous at best.

Exemption is Your Legal Right

Many have the mistaken impression that their children cannot attend public school without "up to date immunizations and vaccinations." This is an untruth. Unless the administration signs that they would personally take responsibility for any possible results, such as learning disabilities, autism, mental retardation, respiratory allergies, and of course death, just to name a few of the possible side effects, there is no reason that your child cannot attend school or college without immunization. Every state has a waiver for legal exclusion from immunization requirements.

It is your legal, and/or religious right to conscientiously object to immunizations and vaccinations. Most states have a form which can be obtained from your public

Authentic Health

health office which states this. Any parent can refuse this "service" for their child and be allowed other public services, such as education. The form also states that if there is an outbreak of any of these diseases that your child will be sent home from school. This is rather comical since you probably would not wish your child to be in an environment that is infected or contagious anyway.

I am also not in favor of forced exposure to any disease; chicken pox for example. As a child both of my younger siblings contracted chicken pox, which is another form of the herpes virus. Chicken pox is a dying virus. What I mean by a dying virus is that it is another virus that humans have over a course of decades developed a natural immunity. This is as God intended. And the great pharmaceutical giants have decided to capitalize on God's natural provision by developing a toxic vaccine as we develop our own immunity. Then of course they will take credit for the future "disappearance" of the chicken pox. Just like Polio though, eventually no one will get the disease without having taken the vaccine. Yes, you heard me correctly. No one gets polio these days unless they have had the vaccine. The polio disease was dying as the vaccine was introduced; those who survived the vaccine probably already had developed immunity. However, those who took the vaccine and developed polio had no natural immunity and therefore simply contracted the disease from the vaccine.

Unlike when I was a child, chicken pox was not heard of as frequently when I became an adult. However, it is now making a re-appearance as the vaccine is currently part of allopathic medicinal protocol for childhood vaccines regiment.

When my children were little, I used to hear of a parent's child having chicken pox, I would later learn that they had either just had their "shot" for it or that they had attended a birthday party and now two weeks later are getting what someone else already had and gave them at the party. Yes, it was their present to take home and enjoy weeks after the party was over. How did they get it? They ate all that sugar and zapped their immune system, which then could not defend against attack; they were then exposed while in a weakened immune state. Sad, but true; this is how it works. Sugar is one of our weaknesses that will break down our defenses against things that can cross the barrier of our immune shields.

Other options besides Vaccines

At this point you are wondering, if immunizations are not the answer, what is? First nurse your child for at least the first year. This gives your child the immune matrix that he needs. If you were not nursed, take Colostrum with Immune Factors throughout pregnancy in order to establish your own immune matrix that he/she needs in order to pass this vital information on to your child; this will also build your immune system.

What if your child is past nursing? Take Immune Stimulator, which contains colostrums and other immune enhancing herbals. This should be used for 3 months at a minimum and can be used indefinitely as a daily support. If the child is under five, I would suggest using 1 capsule three times opened into a bottle, cup of juice or

Authentic Health

applesauce; you will notice changes within 3 days. Many ailments start with poor bowel function, and you will notice this pattern will improve almost immediately. Running noses will improve and overall immune and energy will improve. If the child is over five, use 3 – 10 capsules a day depending on their size. This is also good for adults and can be used during pregnancy, as well.

Homeopathic Remedies can also be used to improve resistance to viral pathogens. (See also chapter on Colds and Flus) If you wish to detoxify from vaccine damage from vaccines taken as a child,, contact me to design a protocol for your unique concerns. Askchena@hotmail.com

Resources List for Further Reading:
White Lies: A Tale of Babies, Vaccines, and Deception by Sarah Collins Honenberger.
What every parent should know about childhood immunizations by Jamie Murphy
The Sanctity of Human Blood : Vaccination is Not Immunization by Tim O'Shea
The Great HPV Vaccine Hoax by Mike Adams
The Chickenpox Vaccine: A new epidemic of disease and corruption by Mike Orrin
Evidence of Harm: Mercury in Vaccines and the Autism Epidemic: A Medical Controversy by David Kirby
Vaccine Safety Manual for concerned families and Health Practitioners by Neil Miller
What your doctor may not tell you about childhood vaccinations by Stephanie Cave

Authentic Health

The following books are all authored by Harris L Coulter Ph.D.:

<u>A Shot In the Dark Childhood Vaccinations and Juvenile-Onset (Type-1) Diabetes</u>

<u>Vaccination and Violent Crime</u>

<u>Critique of government funded studies</u>

<u>SIDS and Seizures</u>

<u>Do Vaccines Cause Cot Deaths?</u>

<u>Vaccination, Social Violence, and Criminality : The Medical Assault on the American Brain</u>

This is not an exhaustive list. Please invest in educating yourself to make the best choices for the safety and long term health of your family.

Chapter 15: Chronic Pain & Solutions

Causes of Unexplained and Chronic Pain

- ✓ Food Triggers
- ✓ Vaccine Triggers
- ✓ Environmental Factors
- ✓ Body Toxins- Let's clean up our act
- ✓ Emotional –Your body never lies

The Causal Factor, starting at the beginning

Finding the cause is the critical element to resolving the effects of chronic pain. Without addressing the root cause of pain, we never really resolve or eliminate the issue. When we discover and address correctly the cause of the pain, the body no longer has to continually fight an unknown enemy. The unknown is often more frightening than the known and understood.

One of the first factors to investigate is food triggers. As we've discussed before food reactivity is usually one of the most foundational areas we leave unaddressed in our modern approach to health. Discovering your food reactivity levels, particularly to common foods you eat regularly, will help you resolve these allergic responses

Authentic Health

and eliminate chronic pain which is triggered by these foods becoming a toxin, when they are not completely digested. Common foods, which often trigger chronic pain or foods which contain oxalic acid are the following (in decreasing order):

1. Buckwheat
2. Star Fruit (Carambola)
3. Black Pepper
4. Parsley
5. Poppy Seed
6. Rhubarb
7. Spinach
8. Chard
9. Beets And Beet Greens
10. Banana
11. Cocoa
12. Chocolate
13. Most Nuts
14. Most Berries
15. Bean

These foods bind with calcium foods to form what are essentially stones. These can form within the kidneys, especially stones formed from oxalic acid which is a kidney irritant. Symptoms of such conditions as gout, osteoporosis, rheumatoid arthritis and kidney disorders are greatly increased when consuming these foods. Tea and coffee also contain small amounts of this offensive chemical therefore avoiding these substances will allow the body to heal and recover faster.

Besides such chemicals as oxalic acid, most any food can become a toxin, when under digested and over-consumed. A food reactivity analysis should be performed in order to determine what other foods may be toxifying your body by inhibiting the healing process of your body. Once these are addressed the healing process will begin to speed dramatically.

In addition, foods from the night shade family, such as tomatoes, potatoes, and eggplants all contain chemicals which cause inflammatory response. Eliminating or reducing these foods within your daily diet will greatly reduce inflammatory response and consequently reduce pain.

I would like to differentiate between chronic pain induced by foods listed above. The above foods contain specific chemicals which will trigger the body's pain mechanisms. This is different than a food allergen, like wheat or gluten intolerance. With intolerances, foods that might otherwise cause no problem become toxic due to an inability to digest them completely. In contrast the foods listed above contain a chemical which when present in body tissues causes pain.

Vaccine Triggers

Often a vaccine from the past as far back as childhood may be a significant causal factor to consider. Polio is a disease causes paralysis as well as other health challenges. People taking the vaccine occasionally have the manifestation of polio even though they were formerly healthy individuals. Thus, today the vaccine intended to enable individuals to avoid polio actually causes the polio itself. The disease introduced by the vaccine may also be a trigger factor in such diseases as fibromyalgia and chronic fatigue syndrome. For this reason, vaccines are likely to be a trigger factor for other modern diseases, as most people today have received the polio vaccine. In addition, many of the ingredients contained in current vaccines are known neuro-toxins and heavy metals. Heavy metals will bind with calcium in particular. When calcium is bound, the pain threshold of the body decreases. This means that the body will feel pain at lower levels of stimuli. In contrast, when high levels of calcium are present, the body does not react to pain in the same manner or does not acknowledge it at all.

For those people who are experiencing long-term chronic pain, simple vaccine detox protocol may be all that is necessary. Strategic supplementation to eliminate and reduce their daily pain levels should also be taken. This protocol would include such supplements as Bentonite Clay , along with specific homeopathic remedies unique to the individual's symptoms. I am happy to provide these personalized homeopathic remedy or detoxification protocols. (You may contact me via email at askchena@hotmail.com or via facebook to receive your homeopathic or protocol for detoxification.) Along with the homeopathic preparation will come a specific protocol, unique to the individual. You may contact me by email with details of your condition and I will tell counsel you on how I can help with this detoxification process. Detoxification may also be extraordinarily helpful with ADD and other personality disorders, as well as autism.

Environmental Stress Factors

Environmental stress factors such as geopathic stress can be caused by such things as overhead wires. Electrical and telephone wires running overhead or over your home while you sleep and rest can be a significant factor in poor long term health. Specific diseases which are likely triggered and continued by geopathic stress factors are arthritis and cancer. If you are dealing with long-term pain situations, which involve either of these extreme conditions, it would be important to have your house, in particular your bedroom laid out to adjust for geographic stress factors present in the room. You can do research online to find a method for detecting geopathic stress and creating a peaceful healing home environment.

If you live in or near a sub-station for electrical power plants, it is likely that you have geopathic stress affecting your health. If you have significant water bodies, such as underground springs or streams running under your home, these are likely to create a situation where geographic stress negatively affects your body. Something as simple as relocating the positioning of your bed or other furniture within the bedroom could be all that is necessary to see significant reduction in pain levels.

Other environmental stress factor can be such things as: new carpet, old carpet, dirty ductwork, mold, asbestos, or formaldehyde within building materials. These environmental factors can also trigger daily pain and continued stress on the body of some individuals.

Body Detoxification

It is important to recognize that daily consumption of foods and substances that your body cannot completely process will over time become toxins in the body. This is because the body is unable to process them out and eliminate the waste, they have produced. When this occurs, the body becomes heavily toxic and in need of detoxification.

In order to detoxify, it is important that the bowels, skin, liver, lungs and kidneys be addressed. EnviroDetox is a formula specifically designed to help detoxify all of these eliminatory channels. Along with EnviroDetox, use Bentonite Clay (1 tablespoon twice daily), these will aid the body greatly in gradually removing toxic substances and eliminate the stress, they are causing. Once these toxins are removed the toxic burden load will greatly diminish, and over time a pain free body will result.

It is important that the bowels remain properly functioning during this time, as most toxins will more readily be eliminated through the bowel than through any other eliminatory channel. If hives should manifest, it is likely that the skin and kidney need extra support during the detoxification period. The herbs Yellowdock and Dandelion may be specifically beneficial in this case.

Once detoxification has begun, the body should steadily begin to improve. Chronic pain levels will reduce; healing will begin to manifest. For specific protocols to detoxify, contact me by email for an individual plan for your unique recovery process.

Authentic Health

The Emotional Connection—Your body never lies

Have you ever been asked, "How are you doing?" Only to lie politely and say,"I'm fine." Though it is an inconvenient truth, your body cannot lie, even though your mouth will; the body is always communicating with you and for you. It is your first advocate in health. We must as a society learn to listen and hear what our bodies are saying and stop taking an Advil to put it in its place and repress the obvious for later. In Carol Truman's book, <u>Feelings Buried Alive Never Die</u>, she explains the connection of the physical pain and sickness we experience and the emotions we lock or bury in our mind. Just like a rotting piece of food in the cabinet, though it is unseen, the stink will eventually be experienced.

"We CAN change our thoughts and this CAN change our feelings and our actions. However, if the thoughts are caused by unresolved deep-seeded feelings that are governing our existence, the thoughts will reoccur time and time again unless we resolve the core feeling."

It becomes our necessity to uncover the offense and allow ourselves with God's assistance to forgive and move past that broken moment in time. We must accept that moment as "a part of our story" and not a part of our victimization; a place where we grow from not a place that defines who we are now. The how becomes the difficult part in this. Many people are in need of an intuitive counselor to guide them through to arrive at this healing moment.

Personally, I experienced a season when I could not breathe well at night. I could breathe fine throughout the day; but as soon as I lay down, I began to wheeze and couldn't get a satisfying breath. In fact it was painful to even try to breathe. This went on for several weeks, until I realized the emotional trigger that had begun the whole thing. Once unveiled, I was able to address the situation with the person who had instigated this sensation. I experienced immediate relief and never experienced that again.

It is not always a new offense and sometimes requires a deeper emotional healing session to unearth the buried experiences of childhood. For example, following the birth of my second child, Felicia, also my first daughter, I began to have irrational fears that someone would attempt to molest or abuse her. I refused to leave her alone with anyone except my mom or grandmother even for a very short time. For several months I did not discuss these feelings with anyone because on an intellectual level I knew that the strength of these feelings was beyond reason.

I began reading the book I mentioned above and began to ask God for revelation in the origin of this fear. The memory of a childhood molestation by a relative came to me. I was a very small child and remembered who, where and under what circumstances. With this memory, I was able to talk to my husband, mother and relieve myself of the burden of carrying that alone. Once it was out, I was also able to forgive that person. I realize that my story sounds over simplified, however, with the help of God and the book I had begun reading just in the season when that information would be most valuable, I was able to be healed and move forward empowered to help others. The philosophy I live by is "acid only destroys the

Authentic Health

vessel that carries it." I am the vessel, I do not have to choose to carry the acid once it has been discovered.

Some people need to forgive themselves or others. This seed of unforgiveness begins to take root and then destroy the mind, body and spirit little by little. The health of the body bears witness to the seed of unforgiveness. I have come to believe that everything that has happened in my life, though much was unpleasant, has allowed me to speak to the pain others are experiencing and help them move from a place of pain and into a place of comfort and peace and more importantly a place of empowerment. In this place you begin to believe that everything can indeed be used for your good and the good of humanity; your personal suffering can have meaning and purpose.

I counsel people body, mind and spirit; as the three are so intricately connected, they manifest in the natural world first in our thoughts then in our health or dis-ease. God has given me an ability to see into a person's health and see causal factors even when the person does not divulge this information. In this way He allows me to speak into their life and if allowed to bring true inner and outer healing. Scriptures teach us: Beloved, I pray that you may prosper in all things and be in health, just as your soul prospers.--3 John 2. Your health is a manifestation or physical proof of your soul's condition. When we suffer outwardly, there exists within us something that our soul has not dealt with or has been unable to resolve. Our body is begging us to find peace and resolution.

Authentic Health

I make myself available as an intuitive healer and will work with people who are suffering to find their place of health and prosperous, productive living no matter where they reside. My contact information is listed at the close of this book.

As an intuitive healer, I allow the Holy Spirit to assist me in finding the core issue which is impacting an individual's lack of health and vitality. Through this unusual gift, Christ allows me the opportunity to serve mankind and share the peace and healing of body, mind and spirit which He desires all of us to enjoy.

I live by 3 John 2 which states, "Beloved, I wish above all things that thou mayest prosper and be in health, even as thy soul prospereth". Our physical health is significantly affected by our spiritual condition and therefore we need to address more than just the physical, especially with a chronic health issue.

Authentic Health

Chapter 16: Everyday Pain

Understanding what the sign posts are saying when you feel pain

✓ Learn the difference between hot and cold fevers
✓ Key Recovery Strategies- Assisting the body to Heal
✓ Homeopathics for Faster Recovery

Pain is only a Sign Post

Pain is an interesting sensation. If you consider that pain is better than the alternative of death, it takes on a whole new meaning. Pain is the body's way of letting us know we need to adjust course. If we don't want to continue having pain, we seek to discover the origin or cause of the pain. Once we discover the source, we are empowered to change course and change the outcome. We can recover from pain. Our bodies are God-designed to repair themselves.

Headaches: Many Causes, Many Solutions

When the body feels pain like a headache, the first question you might ask is, "what is causing this pain?" Blood vessels may constrict and tighten or they can expand and feel intense pressure. Either discomfort is triggered by a singular source. That source is a weakened functioning liver. The liver ceases to send the proper

Authentic Health

histamine levels to keep blood vessel pressure normalized. In essence the culprit in causing the pain is actually the liver. In the case of pain, a secondary partner can be the adrenals. When adrenaline and cortisol levels are not correctly balanced blood flow is inhibited, thus the brain sends messages of intense pressure. By cleansing the liver and supporting the adrenal glands, the body will begin to produce balanced levels of energy, as well as eliminate the painful headaches altogether.

It is important to be able to detect the outward signs from a young child who cannot communicate the sign posts. This will allow you to identify the problem before it escalates into a crisis. Common signals displayed by children are the following: holding their head with their hands, looking downward away from light or downward with hopes of reducing pressure build up, and/or dark circles appearing beneath the eyes. Constipation will also usually be a sign. Given these, it is important to stimulate the liver to produce a bowel movement.

Sometimes an enema will be necessary to get ahead of the headache. A small dose of a teaspoon of Castor oil, or a tablespoon of Liquid Cleanse will move the bowels to eliminate the pain causing element. Cleansing supplements are especially necessary if you notice the signs following an unfortunate diet full of junk foods.

Once bowels are considered (as this is your most likely cause) look at the functioning of the liver. Headaches that are felt behind the right eye are triggered by toxicity lodged in the liver. Cleanse the liver with herbal blends like Milk Thistle Combination and/or Chinese Liver Cleanse. These will speed the body's cleansing process

Authentic Health

and relieve stress that is triggering the head ache! That is exactly what the liver is saying through the pain.

Another type of headache pain is caused by the thyroid. These headaches uniquely begin in the shoulders, work their way up the back of neck and settle on the top of the head. The simplest solution to these is to feed the thyroid. By using Black Walnut, Spirulina, or Thyroid Activator you can begin to feed the suffering thyroid. Once the thyroid gets a consistent iodine rich diet, the body will cease to manifest these painful headaches.

A glandular or hormonal headache begins with a sensation of extreme pressure as if on the edge of an explosion. The sufferer often wishes to make a whole in the top of their head. Black Cohosh will aid in the relief of this type of headache. This type of headache also tends to travel with depression as a companion. Black Cohosh will also take care of the dark mood as well.

The final type of head ache is a sinus headache, these are obvious because they radiate up the nose and above the eyes, like an antenna branching out above the eyes. These headaches can easily be eliminated or managed with Sinus Support and Histablock. These can be taken as needed for occasional suffering or used as a sinus cleanser before seasonal attacks begin. This will clear the congestion that causes this type of problem to occur. It will also enable the body to breathe more freely and clear the congestion itself.

Authentic Health

Stomach Pain

Pain comes in other forms as well, not just headaches. Stomach or abdominal pain is very common in young children. Often it is simply undigested matter and/or parasites. Yes, I said parasites. Constant nagging pain in the stomach is often a sign of fluke worms or other intestinal parasites. Reflux is a typical indication of a fluke worm, and in this case start a parasite cleanse as soon as possible.

To cleanse these worms out, have the child take Black Walnut for several days in high doses. Then begin taking Capsicum capsules at bedtime. Usually within a day or so these worms will be thrown up. They look very much like a large concord grape and appear to have a smooth coat much like a short-haired dog. You will be able to see them when they leave. The first time I threw one up, it crawled down the sink while I stood watching in shock. Once these worms are eliminated digestive discomfort and pain will end.

There are many types of parasites. Don't be surprised at what you might see. You can go online to identify them if you want to know who's been free-loading on your meals. In cases where you suspect you have been dealing with parasites for an extended time, use Black Walnut with Herbal Pumpkin.

In the case of parasitic infestation, which happens more frequently than any of us would like to admit, we need to understand that several concurrent factors triggered the continuation of their survival. First, low enzyme function; second, poor pH balance, and third, low intestinal flora, in

Authentic Health

order to solve these issues use the following protocol along with anti-parasitic herbal mixtures listed above. Following the resolution of these issues continue the protocol below in order to maintain proper digestive health to prevent future issues.

Cause –Source of Problem	Solutions
1. Low Enzymes Production Enzymes/Proactazyme	Food
2. pH Imbalance	Skeletal Strength
3. Low Beneficial Flora	Probiotic 11

Stomach aches are probably the worst thing a mom has to deal with. However, there is a simple solution to these situations.

It is important to discover the cause of the trouble in order to address it most effectively. But to give relief first, use Bentonite Clay for stomach aches. One tablespoon in water or juice will begin to settle the stomach and soak up the cause of the upset. It is possible that there will still be some vomiting as the virus or food poisons may need to leave. However, the Bentonite will work quickly.

Another element to consider is Slippery Elm given in powder or capsule form. Slippery Elm will go into the system and absorb the toxins as well as sooth the membranes which are hot and irritated due to the sickness.

Authentic Health

I have used Bentonite on little children and elderly folks. It is tried and true and can also be used on animals that are vomiting for no apparent reason. It is safe during pregnancy and nursing.

Gallbladder Attack

A gallbladder attack is characterized by extreme pain in the back on your right side. It will manifest below the right breast area about the space of your hand placed below the breast over the rib cage. It will begin in the back of the body opposite where your hand was placed. Many people mistake the pain for a back issue.

People who have this type of pain can get relief from a laying on of hands method, where someone else lays hands over the area front and back. This method requires two hands and that the person with the attack as well as the person rendering aid sit quietly for 20-30 minutes with hands in place while the attack settles down.

While this method will help with the pain, it does not solve the actual problem of a gall bladder that desperately needs to be cleansed.

The following is a protocol to accomplish this task:

This is a 3 day cleanse.

Day 1: Eat only apple or pear. Drink only apple Juice, Pear Juice or water.

Take Cascara Sagrada 2 capsules three times daily.

Take Hydrangea and Gall Bladder Formula 2 capsules of each 4 times through the day.

Day 2: Continue to only eat or drink apple or pear.

Continue taking above supplements at the above dosages.

At bed time make a slushy of ice, 4 ounces of lemon juice and 4 ounces of olive oil. Drink through a straw. Then lie on your right side and sleep.

Day 3: Your stones will likely pass this morning. Continue the above recommendations for eating and drinking and supplements, as more stones will likely to pass throughout the day.

Day 4: Eat broth soups and mild foods as you ease your digestive system back into a more normal diet.

Appendicitis

The pain of appendicitis originates in a clogged bowel. For this reason it is important to keep bowels functioning in good daily working order. Three or more eliminations daily is healthy function anything less is insufficient for the American diet.

If pain occurs in the abdominal cavity as a sharp knifing pain, that seems to travel. It is possible that the appendix is in trouble. Immediately begin the following:

LBS II 1 capsule hourly during waking hours until bowels begin to move.

Silver Shield 1 Tablespoon hourly, as the appendix is full of infection when it ruptures and you are attempting to clear the body of infectious matter.

Lymphomax 2 capsule hourly, as the appendix acts as a cleansing organ for the lymph as well as the bowel and can become overloaded. This will help clear the lymph.

Also if bowels have not been moving regularly, do an enema as this make give you immediately relief and allow you to begin the protocol and get your body normalized.

If the body spikes a fever this is another indicator when coupled with the roving pain, that the appendix may be in crisis. If pain becomes unbearable and you have had no relief from the supplements, this is one of the rare situations when you must head to the hospital.

If surgery is necessary, you will want to follow the protocol to cleanse the vicious toxins from your body, as well as, take Probiotic 11- 4 capsules twice daily to clear yeast and fungus which your system is flooded with due to antibiotics the hospital will give.

Groin Pain

Sharp pains in the groin are often connected with poor bowel functions. This can lead to herniations in the groin, most common on the left side of the body. These are typically along the crease of the inner thigh. This type of stress can become a crisis if left unchecked. At the first sign, (which might appear like a swelling or protrusion out of the abdominal wall) you should begin anti parasitic remedies, such as Black Walnut, Pau D' Arco, as well as

Authentic Health

astringent herbs like Red Raspberry and White Oak bark. These will clear out parasites along with toning, strengthening and tightening the bowel wall. Otherwise, the long term consequence is that the bowel will slip through the tear in the wall. Once this happens, the tear will close up pinching off the portion of the bowel which has penetrated the break in the wall. This can not only be painful but possibly life-threatening.

The only medical solution is surgery. In order to prevent the necessity of this, watch for signs of such a difficulty. Ultimately, this condition is caused by high yeast (a fungal parasite) levels. This can occur when a person eats large quantities of bread, carbohydrates. The gases inside ferment and expand, putting continual pressure on the bowel wall, and eventually breaking down the integrity of the abdominal wall. To prevent this situation, use Probiotic 11- a friendly flora and Food Enzymes. Also, lessening consumption of these foods will be helpful. How much do you desire the abdominal wall to expand enough to pop? Sounds painful, and it is!

When my husband and I were newly married, I noticed that he appeared to have a third testicular sac. Since it had not always been present, I mentioned this to him, thinking he had lifted and strained himself on a previous occasion. He responded that it had been there in the army and they called it a hydrocele (water sac) and said as long as it didn't hurt, not to worry about it.

It remained part of the family through 3 more children. Approximately 5 years later, instigated by a ton of homemade bread for which we proudly ground the wheat and made fresh daily, he had an excruciatingly painful flare up. Everyone we knew pronounced its solution to be surgical and no other alternative. My husband did not agree. He began taking high doses of PauD'Arco and White Oak bark. Within days the inflammation and pain was eliminated. He has since never had a painful flare up. However, he is very conscious to keep bread consumption to a low level and if he feels the slightest uncomfortable feeling coming as before, he immediately begins the protocol again. (He has used these supplements occasionally about 3 times in 14 years.) However, he did take them for months during the first occasion to completely heal and repair the groin and abdominal muscles and kill off the yeast.

Chapter 17: Fevers

Understanding that a Fever IS a sign of health

✓ Learn the difference between hot and cold fevers
✓ Key Recovery Strategies- Assisting the body to Heal
✓ Homeopathics for Faster Recovery

Every Mother's First Nightmare

Let's take just a moment to understand that a fever is a sign of health. Yes, health. The body that is cold is dead. So, if the body can make a fever it is a sign that the body has the ability to heal. Heat is life. We must begin to shift our thinking beyond the current misinformation promoted through the television and other media. The way to wellness is not a purple pill or children's Tylenol. The way to wellness is assisting the body in getting back to balance.

Most mother's begin motherhood without considering what lies ahead in the roller coaster of parenting. One of the first such traumas is usually the first fever.

Our son began his first fever one fine October day. We were sure the fever was high because he felt so hot and seemed so uncomfortable. I don't believe in the thermometers any longer as they simply confirm what you already know to be true. Doctors use them only to alarm and frighten. Anyone can tell when their child's temperature has elevated by touch. You should also check the feet, as cold fevers often have cold feet, conversely hot fevers will have hot feet.

Since we had no intention of giving Tylenol or any other drug option to bring the fever down we needed a better understanding of what the body was trying to accomplish. It is our belief is that the fever occurs naturally in order to bring about a healthy body response to an attack. This is normal, healthy and natural. Our bodies are designed that way by God. By taking drugs that suppress symptoms, you actually inhibit or slow the process of recuperation and healing. Pain medications also work in that manner. These drugs slow your recovery. How often do you hear of a child that took Tylenol every night to reduce a fever that seemed to reappear every time Tylenol wore off. Perhaps they should ask "what is this body trying to burn off?" With this understanding your body can, with the aid of common sense, throw out the "dis-ease" it is fighting.

The best and most speedy method to deal with a fever is to support the body's ability to throw off the fever. The fever itself is not the problem; it is only a signal of a larger attack which the body must fight. We must assist in the success of this attack.

Is this a hot or cold fever?

How do you know the difference? It is simple. First, think about what you are observing. You are probably wondering at the fact that there is more than one type of fever. Yes, in fact there are two types of fevers both requiring different responses to aid in their departure.

Authentic Health

Though the body manifest external heat that is measurable by a thermometer, the internal heat may not be consistent throughout the body thus causing a lingering sickness.

Hot Fevers

The first type of fever is a hot fever. This means that not only is the body hot, but the person is aware of their increase in body temperature. If you are observing an infant for example, they will be throwing off their covers and will wants to drink cool water. A cool cloth will help sooth them and light sheets or blankets will be more comforting than a heavy blanket or quilt. This type of fever must be kept under control but needs to be broken.

The first thing to understand is that you can control the fever without drug therapy. By simply soaking the child or adult in a hot bath you can aid the body in throwing off the fever. Hot water will not feel scalding to the hot fever but rather soothing. Next, put a cup of apple cider vinegar into the bath. This will open the pores of the body and allow heat to escape, lowering the fever. This method of hydrotherapy will also keep the sick person from dehydrating as the body is able to absorb water through the skin. People ask how long they should leave the little one in the bath, the answer is to leave them until they urinate in the tub. This is usually is about 20 minutes. At that point their body has hydrated enough to through off some of the offending toxins.

Our son had a hot fever. I called the midwife who delivered him, and she gave me the above advice. It worked beautifully. He was nine and half months old

Authentic Health

and was teething. The fever lasted off and on until the teeth arrived two days later. (See section on teething in a previous chapter.) With this type of fever, or with teething, I always sleep with the child in our bed and keep a little basin of water and vinegar next to the bed. Each time the fever peaks and the child becomes restless, I bathe the child from head to toe with the vinegar and water. The fever diminishes and the child is able to sleep again. I always tell people that by the next morning the child smells like a pickle but they feel much better.

Cold Fevers

The second type of fever is a cold fever. This occurs when the body feels hot but the person feels cold, shivery and cannot seem to get warm enough. Most often this is a viral fever.

To aid the body in quick recovery from this fever, a hot bath <u>without</u> the vinegar will be most helpful. You can also take the herb Yarrow or Ginger in tea or capsule, as well as the combination VS-C or CC-A. These help the body to recover quickly from a viral attack. Hot teas like Chamomile are also nourishing and soothing. For a child, Catnip & Fennel in liquid form added to warm water can also be soothing. When the person comes out of the hot bath, have hot towels out of the dryer to wrap them in and put them in a warm bed with lots of blankets.

The purpose of the hot baths in both cases is to break the fever and keep the body hydrated. When the body is heated through hydrotherapy, it enables the body to match internal and external temperatures. When the two are the same the fever can break. The cold fever will linger until the internal temperature matches external temperature. Viruses die from heat. A fever is the body's way of destroying a viral attacker.

Usually, by repeating the hot baths a few times throughout the day the fever will break by the evening. In our home we have rarely had sickness last more than 6 hours at the top end. By using these common sense techniques we have kept our children well for the past 14 plus years.

Remember to get pure water into them as often as they are able. If it is a child remember that they can absorb water through their skin. You will know when they are hydrated because after 10-20 minutes they will urinate in the water. Watch for this while they soak. This will keep them from dehydrating while working through their fever.

Fever Keys

- Have apple cider vinegar in cabinet
- Have a place to take hot baths
- Have VS-C for viral infections
- Have Silver Shield to clear viral DNA
- Ginger Tea to warm and burn off fever

Homeopathy for Fever

Aconite: is for congestion and chill preceding inflammatory fever. Frequent chilliness. Redness of the face, heat and an outward pressing headache. Mental symptoms include: anxiety, and restlessness from the violent circulatory storm. There is dry skin, violent thirst, full bounding frequent pulse and sweating brings relief. If fever is brought on by exposure to dry cold winds or chilling of the body after overheat, especially when warm and sweaty aconite is indicated. It suits the young and robust and has no relation to the weak and sickly. Mental anguish is always a part of the fever. The attack of fever often ends with a fever breaking sweat.

Gelsemium: The person will be dizzy and drowsy, the chill is partial; These types of fevers are brought on by warm, relaxing weather. The fever is accompanied by languor, muscular weakness and a desire for absolute rest and is unaccompanied by thirst.

Sulphur An excellent fever remedy, it comes in after Aconite when the skin is dry and hot and there is no sweat; the fever seems to burn the patient up, and the tongue is dry and red and the patient at first is sleepless and restless, but soon becomes drowsy.

Belladonna: This remedy is marked by being overly sensitive to touch, violent delirium, headache, throbbing carotids and cerebral symptoms. Eyes red and glistering; the skin is hot and burning; the heat seems to steam out from the body; it may be followed by a profuse sweat which brings no relief. General dry heat with chills, little or no thirst, in fact, the patient may have a dread of water, cool extremities and throbbing headache. The fever is worse at night.

Nux vomica This fever is characterized by great heat; the whole body is burning hot, the face is especially red and hot, yet the patient feels chilly when uncovering.

Bryonia Suits especially a quiet form of fever; the person may be restless and toss about, but is always made worse thereby. There is intense headache, dull, stupefying with a sensation as if the head would burst at the temples; manifesting sharp pains over the eyes, faintness on rising up, dry mouth and a tongue coated white in the middle. Cold, chilly sensations predominate in fevers calling for Bryonia, and there is much thirst for large drinks of water at rather infrequent intervals.

Rhus toxicodendron A form of catarrhal fever. It begins with weakness of the whole body with desire to lie down, soreness or bruised sensations in the limbs; aching of limbs and bones; great pain in the back, restlessness; worse while lying still: stomach sickness; loss of appetite and repugnance for food; great thirst; along with a dry tongue and mouth.

Authentic Health

Chapter 18: Colds

Understand the 2 different types of Colds and what they are telling you

✓ Learn the difference between viral and bacterial attack
✓ Key Recovery Strategies- Assisting the body to Heal
✓ Homeopathic Remedy for Faster Recovery

Mother's Winter Battle

Colds are mothers' second battle attacks predominantly in the winter. I know with nine children it seems in the winter someone is always coming down from a night's sleep with a running nose. Keeping watch over this beginning sign of a cold is important and at times can feel impossible.

However, if you know the signs of the different types of colds you can identify the most likely cause and get rid of it as quickly as possible.

Dark circles under the eyes may indicate over consumption of dairy products. Some Bee Pollen sprinkled into applesauce will clear this up quickly. Colds are especially common in the winter months. During the wintry weather we do not consistently consume enough sulfur rich foods. These are important to a healthy digestive system and therefore keep the immune system

Authentic Health

from frequent attack. Garlic and onions are both sulfur rich foods. These can be minced or chopped and hidden in many dishes in order to boost the nutrients that feed the immune system. The chemicals in garlic also feed the good bacteria in your body which help digest foods and fight sickness.

Always keep onions and garlic around. I keep a large jar of minced garlic and lots of onions in the house at all times. The idea of feeding a cold is valid. Hot, spicy, liquid foods like chicken noodle soup, or egg drop soup are best because they warm the body from within and boost natural potassium.

Onions have another use that can turn a cold around. When a cold strikes, try using an onion foot soak. Take an onion diced up and put in to a hot foot soak. This will pull a virus or cold out through the feet. Onions can also be used to draw out infection from the ear, nose, and throat. Take an onion and slice it steak thick bake in the oven until onion is juicy and soft. Then place on a thin cloth, like an old thin tea towel. Place on the throat, ear, or lungs with heat from heating pad, or hot water bottle. Leave on the area until it is no longer hot. This will go through the skin and begin to assist in fighting the infection.

Colds, like fevers, can be different. Look at the signals the body is giving. Is the nose runny? Can you see thick or thin mucous? Is the mucous clear or colored?

Important KEY: *If you see clear mucous, you are looking at a viral infection. However, if you see colored mucous the body is trying to clear a bacterial infection.*

Authentic Health

When a Cold is Viral

Many times the body will begin with a cold that is viral in nature. Silver Shield Liquid could stop this in its tracks. After days of mucous discharge, bacterial infections can settle in and compound the problem. It is best to catch these things in the beginning, but if things go too quickly, it is important to have on hand herbs like Peppermint Oil, Oregon Grape, CBG Extract and Garlic Oil. Having these on hand can help address the respiratory system quickly. Peppermint oil or Tei Fu oil can be used to open respiratory system just by inhaling them. You could also add 3-5 drops into warm water to make a tea. This tea will help soothe the throat and open breathing passages.

When a Cold is Bacterial

Oregon Grape is a wonderful antibiotic that will not affect the good bacteria in the colon. CBG Extract is used as a natural antibiotic and is also great for ear infections and sore throats. Garlic oil taken daily by children can eliminate most sickness. Have your child take 1 capsule daily in the evening. This will keep children's immune systems strong. Most illness will be avoided with this approach. A daily dose of Silver Shield liquid 1 tsp daily can act as a great protector during cold and flu season.

Vitamin C is widely known and respected for cold relief. I prefer a Vitamin C Ascorbates, which is powdered and rapidly absorbed. This form of Vitamin C is put into juice or water and drank. By using a liquid form of C you can get a larger dose in one quick drink. Another source for Vitamin C is not orange juice. While orange juice can contain Vitamin C it is not the highest source of this vital enzyme. The highest source for Vitamin C is pineapple juice. This juice also contains the digestive enzyme bromelain. This enzyme breaks down mucous, a perfect complement to the Vitamin C's ability to boost the immune to fight the common cold.

The Hero is YOU

If parents can grasp the concept that prevention truly serves us better than a heroic medicine. Imagine waiting till the house fall sideways or until the roof leaks to make a decision that you would like a nice house. Take care of the house you have and continue to strategize to improve it. Likewise, your body should be the same. It is much easier to start the body off right than to have to rebuild. If we watch for weakness or stress we can effectively eliminate most sickness. But if we violate the strategy we set forth, we can do nothing but reap the seeds we have sown.

It is frustrating to me to hear of a child that is always sick, or has reoccurring sickness and discover that the parent's have never considered that the McDonald's diet they are feeding them may be the cause. Consider that when you ingest the grease and fats from the French fries you use up the sulfur your body needs to fight colds and infections. If you are prone to sore throats and colds you are probably allergic to fats. You need to reduce the toxic fats in the diet (heated oils) and increase the good sources of sulfur: onions, garlic and strong pungent smelling foods.

Authentic Health

These are common sense foods. During the bubonic plague it was the criminals who survived, having only been fed onions and garlic. The pauper's diet could literally save you and your family from much sickness.

Keys to Treating a Cold

- Onions & garlic always on hand
- Silver Shield liquid in a nasal spray
- Remember 1 capsule of Garlic Oil each evening before bed
- Hot baths help burst a fever and clear a cold
- Have Vitamin C Ascorbates and Pineapple juice on hand
- Get warm from the inside using hot baths or hot foot baths with minced onions to burst fever and clear a cold
- Tei Fu Oil to inhale or massage into the skin will make breathing easier and open the respiratory system and break down congestion.

Homeopathy for Colds

Aconite is used for a barking cough, a burning sore throat, and a bitter taste that lingers in your mouth.

Allium cepa Is used when your runny nose feels as though it burns, your eyes water constantly, and you sneeze often. This is homeopathic red onion. It is recommended if your cold makes you feel even worse than you do when you are chopping a strong onion.

Arsenicum album is indicated if you feel chilly, restless, and weak. This remedy is for the individual who, feels worse in a cold room but wants something cold to drink. You probably have a red nose and runny nasal secretions that burn the nose and upper lip. You generally want to be left alone, but like a bit of attention every once in a while.

Belladonna is called for if there is high fever and a headache.

Bryonia is indicated when the cold has moved into the chest and has become largely a cough.

Dulcamara Is indicated for cold when you are opinionated and uptight and shows the following specific symptoms: brought on by weather changing from hot to cold; profuse, watery discharge from nose and eyes; aggravation from catching a cold; also gets conjunctivitis, diarrhea, cystitis, lower-back pain; hay fever, especially at the end of summer or fall; mucous worse in warm room

Eupatorium Is used when you have a severe aching deep in the bones and a feeling of being sore all over.

Authentic Health

Euphrasia is useful if eyes are the main focus of the cold. Also for symptoms that are the opposite of those calling for Allium cepa. The nose runs a lot, especially in the morning, but without irritation. You complain of burning eyes and stinging tears, wink frequently, and wipe and rub your eyes. You also yawn a lot and prefer to be inside, away from sunlight and bright lights.

Gelsemium is helpful when you have chills, aching arms and legs, and fatigue, or if your throat hurts. Also if you have heavy, droopy eyes; feel weak and tired, with aches and chills up and down your back; and want to be alone.

Ipecac Is especially valuable in treating an infant's bronchitis. Adults can use it for a deep cough that has much accumulation of mucus in the chest.

Kali bichromium is given at the later stages of a cold. It is also good for sinus headaches and blocked sinuses with nasal discharge.

Mercurius solubilis if the cold is accompanied by a sore throat that resists treatment.

Nux vomica is indicated if you feel irritable and have a runny nose that becomes congested at night.

Pulsatilla this remedy is often prescribed if you have a stuffy nose and thick yellow discharge. You feel worse at night, prefer to be outdoors, and want comfort and attention.

Spongia is often used for harsh coughs.

Chapter 19: The Flu

Understand the 2 different types of Flu

- ✓ Learn the benefit of sweat
- ✓ Understand how to alleviate nausea &vomiting
- ✓ Key Recovery Strategies- assisting the body to heal
- ✓ Homeopathic Remedies for faster recovery

The flu is often an unexpected crisis that hits without much warning. You arrive at home to a sick child with nausea and vomiting. They are feverish perhaps, but klhaving chills. Now, the fun begins. You must get rid of the flu before the rest of your household gets it.

Using Sweat Equity to your Body's Advantage

The simplest solution is to sweat it out. Hot teas, like: ginger, chamomile, peppermint and yarrow will help your body to warm up inside. It will help the body activate the digestive system. It will also help the skin to begin to sweat and throw out the virus causing the symptoms. A virus can only be killed by heat. The body needs to burst a fever. If you have one available, a sauna could be very helpful as this will help produce a natural fever. When the body begins to sweat or urinate there is an outlet to release the virus.

Authentic Health

It is important to stay hydrated so that the kidneys can continue to carry out viral debris. If a person is unable to keep water down, remember to soak in the bath. This will prevent dehydration.

With the flu, the faster you can evoke a fever and break the fever, the faster your body will be rid of the sickness.

Nausea & Vomiting

The most effective remedies are Bentonite Clay for the nausea and vomiting. This can be put in water or juice and taken every 15 minutes or every hour.

Also if you are not well equipped in your medicine chest, you can use Peppermint Oil. This essential oil helps stop nausea. Use a drop on the tongue to stop nausea quickly. It is also good for car-motion sickness.

Since the flu is viral in nature, use VS-C to help the body eliminate the virus more quickly. VS-C boosts mineral levels and acts as a natural diuretic and therefore helps the body to clear the virus much more quickly.

Sleep is essential to recovery. If you cannot rest often, you cannot heal as rapidly. It is common that a lack of sleep has actually precipitated the sickness. Rest is critical.

Vomiting is one way the body rids itself of a poison. Lobelia Essence may be beneficial if the person feels that he needs to vomit but is unable to. Take ½ tsp of Lobelia Essence every 15 minutes until the body vomits. (If you need to vomit the virus out; Lobelia will help do so.)

Authentic Health

Must Haves for Flu Season

Bentonite Clay to stop nausea, vomiting, and diarrhea	Take 1 TBSP hourly until well
VS-C to clear virus from the system	Take be the tsp hourly until well
Peppermint oil to settle stomach (should not be used with homeopathics)	Take 1 drop on the tongue as needed
Lobelia to clear the toxin from the body more rapidly	Take ½ tsp in juice or under tongue
Silver Shield to clear virus from the system	Take be the tsp hourly until well

Homeopathy for Flu

Aconite used at the start of a severe illness and fearing death.

Gelsemium this person has a 'bursting' headache, not at all thirsty despite the fever, and feeling very chilly even when the thermometer reading is high. The flu comes on slowly in these cases with deep aching all over.

Eupatorium helps when the person complains that their bones feel broken, and their eyeballs are very sore, along with all the other 'cold-like' symptoms.

Baptisia presents with a very red face, a truly prostrated person, and gastric symptoms.

Oscillococcinium speeds recovery from flu. This remedy is also used for Swine & Avian flu.

Chapter 20: Virus or Bacteria: Knowing the Difference

Understanding your body's message

- ✓ Seeing the different types of mucous
- ✓ Treating a virus
- ✓ Treating a bacterial infection
- ✓ Homeopathic remedies for faster recovery

How is mom to know the difference between a virus that will generally pass out of the system on its own through vomiting or diarrhea and a bacterial infection that may need special herbals to alleviate and aid the body in a speedy healing?

Mucous Makes the Difference

The specific symptom which will give the tell-tale sign is the mucous which the body is producing. Viral mucous looks clear and watery while bacterial infections produce thicker, yellow, green or brown drainage.

In the case of vomiting, viruses are usually the cause. Bentonite Clay will usually absorb intestinal viruses and carry them out of the system while also alleviating the nausea.

Authentic Health

Once you determine whether you are dealing with a virus or bacteria, you can then address it quickly.

How to Treat a Virus

For viral infections, use VS-C. This is a Chinese anti-viral formula which works on herpes, chicken pox, canker sores, cold sores, measles, shingles and intestinal viruses.

Vitamin C is also helpful, along with B-Complex vitamins as these aid in flushing things through the urinary system. This is how the virus will leave your body.

Other helpful foods are: pineapple juice and the ever famous chicken soup with lots of garlic and onions. If the sickness is manifesting in nasal congestion, add a little black pepper. Oregano is also a good antiviral.

How to Relieve the Body of a Bacterial Invader

If however, the infection is a bacterial infection use Vitamin C along with Echinacea, Garlic oil gel caps and Goldenseal or Oregon Grape. I always try to use Goldenseal as a last resort. This herb is currently nearing endangerment due to over harvesting, it is best to use this only when all else has failed. Silver Shield liquid can also be taken hourly and often will eliminate infection very quickly, if taken in high doses. (I have drank an entire bottle in a day during a winter bout with Bronchitis that came on very suddenly.-- I was well the next morning.)

When you see the first signs of yellow mucous, begin using Ultimate Echinacea. This combination brings together the benefits of all three medicinal Echinaceas. It is also a liquid so anyone in the house can take it. Begin taking ½ tsp every hour. If this course of action is consistent at the beginning of symptoms, you will find the sickness relieved within only a few hours.

If the symptoms are not alleviated within a few hours, increase the dosage and add foods such as: garlic, onion, apples, and ginger mentioned earlier. Remember, anytime there is mucous present, all dairy foods should be eliminated. This means, no ice cream, milk, or cheeses. I would not reintroduce these foods again until at least 3 days had passed without any symptoms. Reintroducing mucous causing foods or difficult to digest foods could cause an already weak body to relapse into sickness.

A watchful eye on your part can make the difference between a short illness and a prolonged illness.

With these basics for solving both bacterial and viral infections, you will alleviate most very quickly. However, on occasion you may not catch the problem in time to head off the worst of the infection.

Many years ago my son visited his cousins overnight once during the Christmas holiday. By the next morning, after being around a smoker, eating junk food, staying up later than usual and not drinking enough water, I was looking at a green snotty nose. Yuck! By that point, it was past getting rid of the sickness in a few hours. We were looking at a few days of sickness. This was

Authentic Health

especially rough as we were traveling and at the mercy of our hosts for foods served.

But through consistent efforts of eliminating sweets and dairy and making certain that the bowels were working well, Christian was completely well, shortly after returning home.

We did eventually have to go to a combination called PLS II, which contains Goldenseal, to fight off this infection. Most of his mucous was manifesting in the lungs and head. When infection strikes the lungs, Mullein can be a very good support. I now start him taking Cascara Sagrada in order to keep the bowels functioning well beginning at Thanksgiving and ending after New Years. I also begin during the holiday season supporting the lungs which are his inherent weakness. In doing this, we avoid a lot of discomfort and sickness. By supporting the lungs with a formula called Bronchial Formula and using an adult dosage twice daily as maintenance throughout the winter months he has had no sickness for years now. If he shows signs of illness, beginning I immediately begin hourly doses of two capsules each to avoid sickness getting a foothold.

This preventive approach has kept him well for more than 17 years. Now, in college, he is knowledgeable enough to keep up with his own maintenance program.

Great consistent health does not have to be expensive but it does take some thought, effort, and preparation. The first ingredient is to, again, have a strategy. If you begin with the end in mind, you can daily be empowered to take daily good health to the next level.

Authentic Health

Homeopathics for Symptoms of Infection & Virus

Aconite This remedy is often indicated when fever and inflammation come on suddenly, sometimes after exposure to wind and cold, or after a traumatic experience. The person may be very thirsty and often feels fearful or anxious.

Belladonna Intense heat, redness, swelling, throbbing, and pulsation indicate a need for this remedy. The person's face may be flushed and hot (though hands and feet may be cold) and the eyes are often sensitive to light. Thirst may be lower than expected during fever. Discomfort is worse from motion or jarring, and relieved by cold applications.

Bryonia Feeling worse from even the slightest motion; when ill, the person wants to stay completely still—to be left alone and not interfered with in any way. Fever with chills, a very dry mouth, and thirst are also likely. Tearing pains that feel worse from any motion, but improve from pressure if it adds stability, may accompany local infections.

Calcarea carbonica People who need this remedy tire easily and have low stamina. They tend to feel chilly and sluggish, with clammy hands and feet (though their feet may heat up in bed at night, and their heads may perspire during sleep). Swollen lymph nodes, frequent colds, sore throats, ear infections, and skin eruptions are common. Children who need this remedy are often slow to walk and may have teething problems, frequent colds, and ear infections.

Calendula This remedy is useful as a topical application for cuts, scrapes, and skin eruptions, to prevent and combat infection. It is usually used in unpotentized herbal form, as an ointment or tincture. *Calendula* can also be helpful potentized, when taken internally for boils or infections.

Ferrum phosphoricum This remedy is indicated in the early stages of many inflammatory conditions. It is taken at the very first sign of a cold or sore throat, it often helps a person throw the infection off and not get ill. Fever, pink-flushed cheeks, a general weariness, thirst, and moderate pain and swelling are typical symptoms suggesting *Ferrum phos* in illness or infection.

Graphites A person with unhealthy skin that tends toward cracking, oozing honey-colored discharge, and crusts may benefit from this remedy. Impetigo, herpes simplex, or infections involving the skin around the ears, the eyelids, nose, and sinuses are common—as are tendencies toward recurring colds and earaches. A feeling of sluggishness, slow waking, and difficulty concentrating are other indications for *Graphites*.

Hepar sulphuris calcareum A person who needs this remedy feels extremely sensitive and vulnerable when ill, especially if exposed to cold or drafts. Ear infections, sore throats, sinusitis, bronchitis, and skin eruptions are often seen, and cheesy-smelling discharge or offensive pus may be produced. Areas of inflammation can be very sore and sensitive, and splinter-like pains are often felt (in the tonsils when swallowing, in a boil when the skin is touched, etc.).

Authentic Health

Mercurius solubilis This remedy is needed when a person has swollen lymph nodes, offensive breath, and is extremely sensitive to any change in temperature. A tendency toward night sweats and profuse salivation during sleep are other indications. Infections of the gums, ears, sinuses, throat, & skin often respond to this remedy when the other symptoms fit.

Silica A person who needs this remedy can be sensitive and nervous, with low stamina and poor resistance to infection—leading to swollen lymph nodes, frequent colds, sore throats, tonsillitis, sinusitis, bronchitis, and other illnesses. Boils, easy infection of wounds, and abscessed teeth are often seen. Although very chilly in general, the person often perspires during sleep. Offensive foot sweat with an inclination toward fungal infections is also common.

Sulphur is useful in many kinds of infection where irritation, burning pain, redness of mucous membranes & offensive odors and discharges. Skin problems like: eczema, acne, boils, lymphatic swelling, and inflammation of genitals. Symptoms worsen from warmth & after bathing. Colds, bronchitis, & other illnesses that have been neglected, or infections that drag on.

Chapter 21: The Skin, Eczema, Poison Ivy...etc

Understand that the skin is a reflection of internal health

- ✓ Acne-origins
- ✓ Poison Ivy
- ✓ Eczema and Psoriasis
- ✓ Hives
- ✓ Ring Worm & Athlete's foot or Foot Fungus

Acne

Though many parents believe this condition is a right of passage of a young person; this does not have to be a normal teenage occurrence. It the body's outward expression of an internal imbalance. Acne can have several origins. It can stem from poor bowel, kidney, lung or glandular function.

By observing the location of breakouts and whether they are dry conditions or wet (pus filled) breakouts you can address with the supplement appropriate to the cause listed below:

Authentic Health

Acne Solutions

Location of acne	Origin	Supplement
Forehead	Bowel	Use Bowel Detox
Cheeks/Chest/Back	Lung	Use Bronchial Formula
Chin	Reproductive Glands	Use Mastergland
Other Areas of Body	Kidney	Use Red Clover & Yellowdock

(A more complete visual face diagnosis chart can be ordered: to obtain: contact by email. You can also email a picture of your face for a complete face analysis complete with supplement and lifestyle recommendations for your personal health issues. Email to request this service.)

When you address the origin of the acne, it will clear up more rapidly. Topically you can apply Bentonite Clay as a mask twice a week, and apply Herbal Trim Lotion topically at night to soothe and Silver Shield gel topically in the morning to speed healing.

Poison Ivy

What can you do for poison ivy besides run to the doctor for a steroid? First, let's know that those who are sensitive to poison ivy need to decrease sugar intake and cleanse the blood.

Authentic Health

Cleansing the blood can begin to decrease your sensitivity to the toxic resins. BP-X a blood purification formula can begin this process. Also, you must eliminate the sugars from your diet as the blood is not in the right pH balance.

Next, when exposed to the poison, DO NOT wash the skin with soap, as this breaks the first layer of defense your body has against the poison. Instead put Bentonite Clay in liquid form all over the exposed skin. Let dry and repeat a few times. This will absorb the poisonous resin.

A protocol to address poison ivy/oak/sumac

If Exposed	Apply Bentonite Clay topically
If Rash Appears	Take Bentonite Clay 1 Tbsp hourly
If Itching	Take 1 capsule of Capsicum hourly or as needed
If Swelling becomes Severe	Take SC Formula and Una de Gato 1 capsule each hourly or as needed

I have had a reaction on occasion when a neighbor burned poison ivy and the particles became airborne. My face and arms immediately began to swell, and I could tell it was going to be a battle. I immediately did the above. The swelling began to lessen, and the heat in my face began to decrease within minutes of taking Una de Gato and SC Formula.

Eczema & Psoriasis

These two conditions are actually related. Both eczema and psoriasis relate to poor thyroid function. Eczema will appear like a "hot spot" on an animal. It will be itchy and you will scratch without even realizing it. Then the skin will tear and weep. It is not only an uncomfortable problem but also a painful one. For a little child, use liquid Black Walnut and Flax Seed Oil in liquid. For an adult use Thyroid Activator along with Flax Seed Oil. I suggest doubling the bottle recommendation for the first week, to bring about a quick turn around. These should be used with Irish Moss Lotion as a topical application. The first several applications of Irish Moss Lotion will feel as if the skin is burning. As the skin is like a dessert, it will take several applications before you feel the benefit. However, after the about third application the body will begin to feel and look more subtle.

Psoriasis is characterized not by dry, thin, itchy skin but by a thick scaly appearance usually on the joints. In this situation the skin is unable to completely exfoliate, thus the skin gets a thick scaly crusty look. This is due to a poor thyroid function and blood impurities attempting to leave through the skin. Skin brushing can be helpful. Also, bathing in Patchouli Oil can be helpful, too. All Cell Detox is the best formula for clearing this problem. Also, apply Bentonite Clay, and take 1 tablespoon twice daily internally. An infrared sauna several times weekly can also be very helpful.

Eczema is actually the opposite condition. The skin is unable to reproduce its tissue fast enough. In other words, the body is not able to repair itself in the proper

Authentic Health

timeframe. Thyroid Activator will enable the body to correct this situation within a few days. Also, apply Irish Moss Lotion topically.

Remember, if there is a problem with the skin, then the matrix of the blood supply is also lacking, particularly in sulfur and calcium. These two nutrients are essential to healthy skin and to repair of skin. Always feed the inside and then see the difference on the outside.

Hives

Probably one of the most painful and embarrassing of skin conditions, hives can be triggered by many culprits. Examples of causes are: antibiotics taken even a year before hives present themselves; liver toxicity; over-taxed kidneys, allergic response to food or chemical substances and emotions such as irritation. Emotional irritation can also manifest hives.

When hives appear the above are causal factors to consider. The Bach flower remedy Impatients can be very helpful to alleviating hives triggered by emotional disturbances.

The protocol that follows will also be beneficial in preventing future outbreaks as well as clearing up the current situation.

Authentic Health

Protocol to Cleanse the Vital Eliminatory Organs

To Cleanse always cleanse the liver, kidney and treat inflammation and itching.

Here's how:

Cleanse the Liver and Kidney	Dieter's Cleanse	Clears Environmental toxins
Take Anti-Inflammatory herbs	Chinese IF-C TCM	Reduces inflammation
For Itching	Capsicum	Breaks down heat and stops itching

Chapter 22: Bedwetting & Urinary Tract Infections

Understanding your enemy can save you much suffering

- ✓ Causes of Bedwetting
- ✓ Urinary Tract Infections- Causes and Solutions
- ✓ Homeopathic Remedies for Faster Recovery

What Causes Bedwetting?

Bed wetting is an overwhelming problem for many children in the U.S. Why? Perhaps because we train children during infancy to remain wet in their own waste. They acquire a greater tolerance toward being wet. I suggest this after having observed my fifth child who wore cloth diapers. We noticed that she never cried except when she was wet or hungry. She had no tolerance for wetness. Nor do I as an adult. I feel like in the end she was more anxious to stay dry than lie in urine in the bed later on.

Now aside from the societal issues, there are some dietary issues to address. Bedwetting can be caused by many food allergies. The most common are dairy and fruits such as grapes. We removed all dairy including yogurt from our older two girls' diets and their bedwetting ceased.

Authentic Health

From a physiological standpoint, bedwetting can be from having very over-taxed or weakened adrenal glands. This causes low blood sugar. Licorice Root can help this as well as a high protein snack before bed. Also, regular bed times every night make a big difference. We used to have a wet bed every Thursday morning after a later than usual Wednesday night church service. We sometimes forget how sensitive children can be to changes in their lifestyle. Children need structure. Bedtimes are part of that.

We have also noticed a correlation with food colorings in food or high sugar intake before bed. We have chosen not to put the girls in Pull-Ups when these problems have gone on. This was frustrating to be washing so much laundry. However, I felt the girls would never learn to dislike the wet bed if they were in pull ups that just disguised the situation.

Look at the diet, specific food patterns, food colorings and dyes, and high sugar intake and late hours or a child that stays up late even after in bed. Lastly, it should also be noted that bedwetting is emotionally linked to fear and insecurity. Particularly fear of loss of a parent and or their love. It can be connected with a new home, new job, strife between parents (even if the child is not a witness to the strife; they still sense it). So, reassuring your child of your love and love for your mate is an important area to address if this is an on-going difficulty for your child.

Authentic Health

Homeopathic Remedies to Aid Bedwetting

Belladonna– Recommended for cases of involuntary urination (bedwetting) during sleep, especially for those who frequently wet after midnight and toward the morning, have restless sleep with sudden starts, moaning and screaming in sleep.

Causticum - Also recommended for a sleep related bedwetting, especially for those who wet during the first half of the night, or when coughing or sneezing, or children with allergic reactions to smoked food.

Equisetum – For those with an irritable bladder who has urgent and frequent day and night urinations

Sepia - Recommended for children who wet during the first half of the night.

Sulfur - For bedwetters who love sweets and spices, who are 'hot and sweaty", wetting the bed mostly during the second half of the night.

Urinary Tract Infections

If you suspect a urinary tract infection, try using a tablespoon of apple cider vinegar. This will usually clear it up within a few doses. Also, notice if there are any unusual rashes or redness that might indicate a yeast problem. If you suspect yeast, they will also be complaining of itchiness. Aloe Vera Juice is very helpful with this problem. Remember with yeast to eliminate all fruits and juices especially grapes, peaches, and skinned fruits. Bananas and pealed apples as well as berries tend to be ok. Black Walnut Extract will also help with the Candida imbalance.

Along with making sure the person drinks plenty of water, as dehydration can be the beginning trigger, the following protocol will help clear the problem:

JP-X formula	clears infection by shifting pH creating an environment in which bacteria can no longer flourish nor survive.
Lemon Water	helps keep pH balanced.
Marshmallow	pushes out any bacterial or fungal material & reduces pain.

If the person is plagued with these UTI's monthly, look for a pattern. I have found that often municipal water is treated on a certain monthly schedule and those drinking that water, often manifest a UTI in response to the changes in the water in the same monthly pattern. If you notice this, then begin drinking bottled purified water.

Kidney Stones

This is a major issue for many people and it should be noted that the actual cause is a weakened digestive system and poor calcium metabolism. Over a lifetime, this will manifest in stone formation and the pain and discomfort that follows.

Authentic Health

If you come from a family of stone producers, then you should begin taking PDA (a digestive aid which contains Hydrochloric Acid-the missing element in breaking down stones). Begin now, don't wait until you begin to suffer.

Also begin taking Hydrangea and Marshmallow. These herbs will breakdown the stones as well as lubricate the tissue in order for stones to pass more easily. Hydrangea actually begins to fragment the stones. While Marshmallow acts as a lubricant for the tubes leading out of the kidney and into the bladder. You will have less pain and bleeding when stones actually pass.

Lemon water should be consumed regularly throughout the day as a preventative. In the case of a stone attempting to pass you can also drink heavily lemoned water. You should also take 2 capsules of both Hydrangea and Marshmallow hourly until stone passes out.

Chapter 23: Weight Loss & Keys to Balanced Health

Understanding what the body needs to maintain balance

- ✓ Core Nutrition
- ✓ 7 Keys
- ✓ Appetite control
- ✓ Boosting Metabolism
- ✓ Get Up and Go---NOW!

KEYS TO HEALTHY WEIGHT LOSS

Core Nutrition is essential for health, vitality and weight loss. When core nutrition needs are met the body will naturally return to a state of balance and ideal weight. Using the following protocol for 90 days will enable the body to reach this ideal state.

Authentic Health

Core Nutrition Protocol

By meeting core nutrition needs your body's basic needs are met and healing and balance are easier to find. A basic nutrition protocol follows:

Food Enzymes- to better digest what you are eating
Nature's Three- to add fiber and push out old materials as well as feel full and balance blood sugar levels
Super Omegas-to give the body the needed fats to stop cravings, balance glands, and improve cardiovascular health
Super Supplemental-to give the body key nutrients to improve overall health and vitality
Super Antioxidant- to boost energy and immune function.

However, if you wish to speed the detoxification process and eliminate excess body fat more quickly the following protocol has helped others achieve their goal of healthy weight loss.

Authentic Health

7 Keys to healthy weight loss

Fiber is the body's broom. It sweeps wastes out as well as absorbs fats and toxins from the diet and carries it out of the body so that it is not reabsorbed and stored in the form of fat. Nature's Three or Psyllium Hulls will act as this detoxifying agent.

Carbohydrates are your vital energy sources. These break down into sugar for your brain and energy reserves. A great carbohydrate comes from super foods like Wheat Grass, Barley Grass, Spirulina and other super foods which all have healing potential. These are not your "green beans and peas". These are super healing foods. Ultimate Greenzone is the product I specifically use for this.

Protein acts a blood sugar stabilizer and when eaten in the morning, breaks the fast and sets blood sugar levels so that energy drops are less frequent throughout the day. There are several products which will accomplish this task: Love n Peas- made of white peas; Nutriburn-made from whey protein (specifically for weight loss and appetite control); Syner Protein- made from soy protein.

Fats are essential, not potato chips or French fries, but Essential Fatty Acids. These provide protection for the nervous system, aid in glandular functions and help lubricate the bowel so waste can easily slide out. Without Essential Fats the body will not release bad fats and other systems will suffer as well.

Minerals act as a conduit for electrical energy flow in the body. The lack of various minerals can cause a myriad of cravings. Very low levels of minerals will cause a desire

Authentic Health

for ice; low levels will cause a desire for salty, crunchy foods; low levels of manganese will cause nail biting, just to list a few.

Calcium is necessary as an alkalizer. When the body is in an alkaline state, the body will maintain optimum health and diseases such as cancer cannot gain a foothold.

Antioxidants aid the body in feeling energized and having reserves to fight unseen enemies such as flus or colds.

Authentic Health

Speeding Weight Loss & Health Gain

Blend the following ingredients for a delicious fruit smoothie:

Nature's Three 1 TBSP
Ultimate Green Zone half scoop
Syner Protein or Love n Peas Protein 1 scoop (B & O Blood Types may have faster results with NutriBurn)
Flax Seed Oil 1 TBSP
Chinese Mineral Chi Tonic or Ionic Minerals with Acai 1 Ounce
Coral or Sea Calcium 1 scoop
Thai Go can be used to boost immune function
8 ounces of juice (pineapple or grapefruit are best for weight loss)
1 cup frozen or fresh fruit

Authentic Health

Help for common struggles

There are many common struggles amongst those trying to reclaim their body after weight gain has occurred. Many of these issues and their origins are explained in the following section.

Countering Appetite: How to get control

Keeping the appetite under control is a major key in weight loss. Without proper appetite control we give in to cravings constantly throughout the day; never giving the digestive system a break; never allowing the body to completely process all that it has consumed. To do this, you must gain control over the hypothalamus. A simple solution to balance the hypothalamus while also giving the body a "natural tummy tuck" is to use seven capsules of red raspberry first thing in the morning. This balance is the body's natural craving mechanism, while simultaneously strengthening and tightening the abdominal walls giving the body, a natural tummy tuck.

Boosting Metabolism

Keep your metabolism or energy level up is very important to burning fat as well as maintaining good activity physically. To do this, consider smelling citrus or peppermint. These smells are extremely stimulating to the digestive system as well as to the energy level. Essential oils like Lemon, Red Mandarin and Peppermint are all exciting to the mind and energizing to the body.

Supplements like Metabomax contain these natural stimulants which will improve thermogenesis; the fat burning mechanism in the body. These naturally boost energy, while causing the body to burn fat reserves. It is also important to address the liver's natural functions when one is concerned with weight loss. The liver is the only organ which removes fat from the body by dumping it into the bowel, where it is then eliminated into the toilet.

Excess fats in blood stream or diet

Many overweight individuals also have a fatty liver and therefore need to detoxify the liver. Fat grabbers assist the liver in gentle detoxification and are an excellent supplement to aid the body in eliminating fat that is eaten, while also pulling fat from the bloodstream and carrying it out through the bowel. Helpful foods, which might also stack the odds in your favor with weight loss are such foods as cannellini beans, zucchini, lemons, oranges, grapefruit, and pineapple. All of these foods are fiber rich and digestive aids. Again, curbing appetite and pulling fats from the body.

Get Up and Go!

Most people who complain of the inability to lose weight also complain of a lack of energy. This can be because the body's natural energy producing organs are lacking in strength. Organs such as the stomach, thyroid, and adrenals, or the bowels are no longer working at peak.

Dieters Cleanse is an excellent place to begin addressing the bowel, as well as the glands, which are likely affecting energy levels. Another herbal combination that would greatly benefit the body and encourage weight loss is

Authentic Health

Master Gland formula along with Energ-V. These two together will greatly improve the daily energy level, and therefore give you the get up and go that your body really needs in order to be more active and therefore burn more calories.

For those who lack the ability to sick with things Chinese Blood Build helps tremendously to boost commitment level. Also for those who lack drive all together, Maca is a great booster.

Infrared Saunas can also be extremely beneficial in speeding the process of weight loss. As they burn 600 calories in 30 minutes giving you the benefit of the one hour high energy aerobic workout while simply sitting and reading a magazine. Check your local health clubs to see if they might have such a sauna. Other benefits of this type of sauna include eliminating chronic pain, reducing arthritis, lowering blood pressure, improving cardiovascular function, detoxification, improving skin, helping the pain of chronic fatigue, reducing inflammation of fibromyalgia and eliminating depression.

Authentic Health

Chapter 24: The Home Medicine Chest

Having what you need could save you thousands of $$$$$$$$

- ✓ 7 MUST Haves to keep on hand at ALL times
- ✓ Triage
- ✓ Cuts in stitches
- ✓ Bites and stings
- ✓ Swelling, Allergic Reactions, Hives

The basic home medicine chest includes seven key ingredients.

- Silver shield liquid
- Lobelia essence
- Peppermint oil
- Bentonite Clay
- VS-C
- Silver shield gel
- Tei Fu oil

Authentic Health

These seven items will likely keep you out of the doctor's office 95% of the time.

Silver Shield liquid- this will be used for viral, bacterial and fungal infections. It can be used internally by gargling, swishing and swallowing the liquid. It can also be put in, the ears for no less than 10 minutes at a time to rid the ears of ear infections and swimmers ear. It is effective on staph, strep, pneumonia, as well as viral and fungal infections.

Lobelia Essence- this will be mixed with honey and 10 drops of Tei Fu oil to make a cough syrup that will breakup congestion and help breathe easier if there is a deep cough. It will also be used for such problem as heart attacks, strokes or asthma attacks. It can also be used to stop seizures.

Peppermint Oil this will be used for indigestion, gas and nausea. A single drop on the tongue is all it will take. It can also be used for a colicky baby. Place a drop on your finger and lick it off your own finger and then let the baby suckle on what remains on the finger.

Bentonite Clay this can be taken by the tablespoon in juice or water or straight, this will absorb toxins which cause stomach flu, dysentery, nausea, vomiting and food poisoning. It can also be applied topically to clear up poison ivy was and sumac poison oak and other rashes. It can also be applied topically to bug bites or bee stings.

VS-C this formula is available in liquid for children or a concentrated TCM formula capsule for adults is extremely useful for fighting viral attacks intestinal flu cold. Chickenpox herpes and shingles for child take 1 teaspoon hourly for an adult take one capsule of the of the TCM formula hourly until sickness is eliminated.

Tei Fu Oil- this will be used as follows:

For headaches: Rub it into the temples and the back of the neck.
For congestion: Rub it under the nose or on the chest and back.
For coughing: Rubbed on the bottoms of their feet; then place sock on their feet.
For ear ache: Put a few drops into ear and blow gently to release oils. Also rub along the sides of the neck.
For sore throat: Mix with honey and Lobelia; or simply put a drop on your tongue and inhale deeply.
For bruising and pain relief: Apply topically to bruise.

Silver Shield Gel- this is a topical that makes healing fast, because it fights all the things which inhibit healing of skin and tissue. If there is no inflammation and bacterial growth, healing can take place without battling infection and occurs more quickly and with less scarring or no scarring.

From the following photos you can see why I am so passionate that families have on hand the necessary supplies and supplements to quickly care for the needs of our family when crisis arrives.

Authentic Health

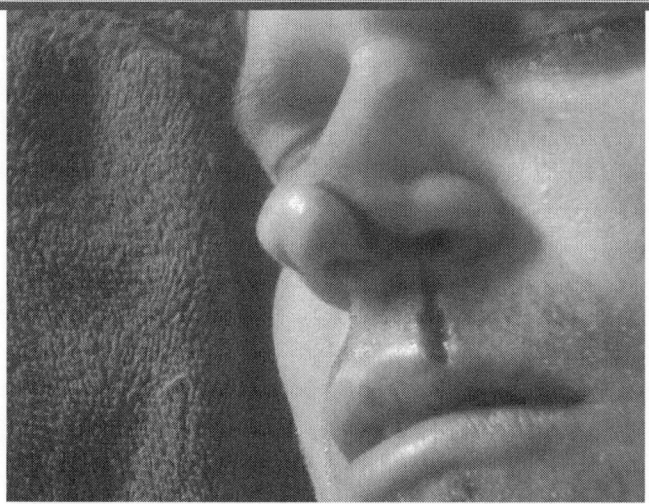

Pictured above is my husband following an accident while working on an engine.

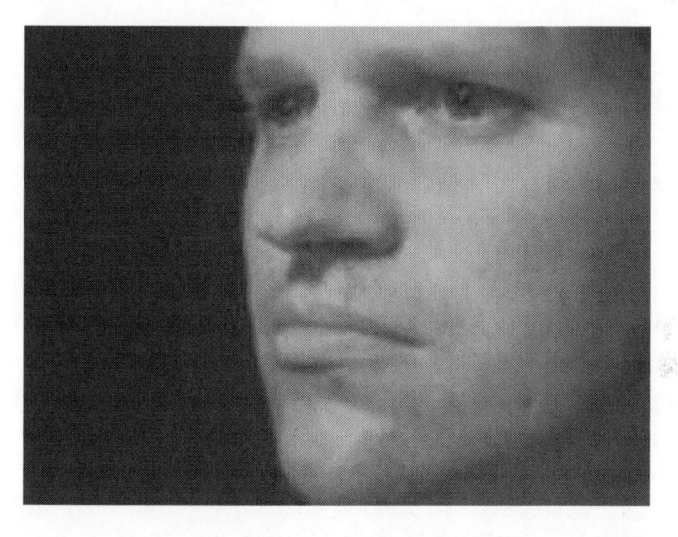

This picture was taken just 5 days later after using Silver Shield liquid and gel. You can just slightly see the scar and today it is barely noticeable at all.

Authentic Health

Quick Answers are as close as Facebook or email
If you have these you will be able to immediately address 95% of all sicknesses that may occur throughout the year. If you're uncertain how much or how often or which supplement or homeopathic is best to use for a given situation you can Facebook message me, CHENA ANDERSON. As these messages come directly into my phone I am able to answer within minutes. If you have more detailed concerns, consulting is available through the internet: send requests to askchena@hotmail.com.

For those purchasing this book who are interested in products such as the homeopathic remedies listed in the book or in testing which has been mentioned previously, you may contact me directly through Facebook or by e-mail at askchena@hotmail.com. Please place the words **Authentic Health** in the subject line. As a gift to those purchasing this book you may also contact me with questions via the above methods as well. If you are sending questions please place **Authentic Health ?** in your subject line.

If you will register your book with me at askchena@hotmail.com, I will send a free gift to your family. To register include email, physical address, and name.

Our family desires to serve through education and consultation. Your free gift will further aid you in achieving Authentic Health and the promise of 3rd 99John 2.

Made in the USA
Middletown, DE
31 January 2015